Indian Medical Science Series No.1

Hindu Practice of Medicine

K.R.L. Gupta

Sri Satguru Publications
A Division of
Indian Books Centre
Delhi, India

Published by
Sri Satguru Publications,
Indological and Oriental Publishers
A Division of
Indian Books Centre
40/5, Shakti Nagar,
Delhi-110007
India

Email: ibcindia@vsnl.com
Website: http://www.indianbookscentre.com

Second Edition ; Delhi, 1986
Reprinted : Delhi, 2001

ISBN 81-7030-091-1

Printed at C vla Offset Printers, Delhi 110 052

Hindu Practice of Medicine

CONTENTS.

PREFACE

"One touch of nature makes the whole world kin
That all with one consent praise new-born gawds
Though they are made and moulded of things past
And give to dust that is a little gilt
More laud than gilt o'erdusted."

Shakespeare.

The compilation of the kind, I have undertaken is still a novel thing in India and if it has been intelligently worked up, I have no manner of doubt that it will meet with the cordial approbation of my kind countrymen. Mere translations cannot now satisfy them. Something in a new form must appear to meet their request. Translations of ancient Hindu medical books have been unnumbered. I myself have had the honour of translating some of the foremost of them. But they are not in touch with the real need of the people. There is much in them that does not stand a careful sifting. We can only come in sight of a few isolated truths after journeying through an enormous mass of rubbish. To help any man to learn useless or spurious knowledge is a crime. Those of the nineteenth century, "when every hour must sweat her sixty minutes to the death" cannot afford to be crammed with what they have no business to remember, while there is so much that they must know, if they are not to be handicapped in the race of life. If we can arrive at the same end by two ways—one short and the other long, the learner ought not to hesitate as to which he should prefer. Moreover those translated volumes are not within the means of every aspirant for Hindu medical lore. India is now absolutely poor and those votaries for Hindu medicine are the poorest of the Indian people. It may be therefore safely hoped that this Hindu Practice of medicine will be appreciated by them yielding as it does—all the gems of the Hindu medical science in one vessel and that for a nominal price. What is best in a Charaka, a Susruta, a Bhabaprakasa or a Baobhat has been thrown into this Hindu Practice of Medicine. It is indeed an epitome of the whole Hindu medical science. To add to its practical utility, I have put in whatever I have found out by my practice which is tolerably long. I sincerely ignore those little jealousies which do not permit Kabirajes to make a public gift of the fruits of their own labour and experience. If the book tends in any way to spread the knowledge of Hindu system of medicine and if it induces my abler fellow workers to make similar publication of their own discoveries, I shall consider my labours very adequately recompensed.

KAVIRAJ R. L. GUPTA.

HINDU

PRACTICE OF MEDICINE

GENERAL TREATMENT OF FEVER.

The treatment of fever varies according as it is new, or has not lasted seven days; is recent, or has not affected the individual more than twelve days; or is old, having continued twenty-one days, or upwards.

When the fever is *new* the patient should only take *conjee* water for food; and when the internal heat is diminished, dry ginger and long-pepper may be boiled in it. When with fever there is a disease in the side, or lower part of the head or abdomen, the red rice should be used for making the *conjee*. Should phlegm be diseased *conjee* should not be given; nor when the new fever is very strong. When these acute symptoms are diminished and when *bile* is deranged the use of *conjee* water is proper. The drink should be boiled water again warmed. Should the patient complain of nausia, and fulness of the stomach, on an accession of fever, the treatment should commence with the exhibition of an emetic, and during the continuance of an attack of fever all heavy food should be carefully avoided; particularly when there is no appetite.

In other MSS. it is stated that the fasting is to be continued for three, five, or ten days, according to the improvement of the symptoms which takes place. By this means the practitioner will discover the state of the air, bile, and phlegm.

During the continuance of a *new* fever the patient should reside in a room shut up, in which a *panká* may be used. He should be clad in warm clothes; should neither sleep during the day, bathe, nor anoint his body with oil. He should also be removed from his wife, avoid all oily and indigestable articles of food, especially astringent articles, anger, violent exercise, and exposure to strong wind. By these means the morbid matter is allowed to ripen, and is then to be discharged by evacuant medicines. It will increase the disease, and render it probably fatal, if these evacuant remedies are used before the morbid matter is matured.

Should in any case the fasting produce weakness, it is to be stopped as improper; and means to strengthen the body substituted. Fasting is not to be employed in fevers which attacks infants or old people, in pregnancy, when the body is light, or in cases in which air, urine, and dejections have been discharged, in large quantities, by medicine.

In recent fever the patient is to be allowed a decoction of bitter herbs, &c. so as to restore the derangement of the humours. He may now be allowed a little more food than during the first stage. Milk, which during the first stage is like poison, may now be taken with advantage.

Should the disease continue and pass on to the third period, when the fever is said to be *old*, it is to be treated by emetics, purgatives, and different febrifuge decoctions. The diet should be in larger quantities and of a more nourishing quality, than during the two first periods of the disease; such as broths, prepared with animal flesh, milk, and the like.

In all such cases of fever it is necessary to recollect that the treatment will vary according as the air, bile, and phlegm are more or less affected.

The fever is said to have disappeared when the appetite returns; the body feels light, and the person is not easily fatigued. When the acuteness of his senses, memory, and understanding is restored, the unnatural heat of the body disappears, and he has no pain; when he moans, is forgetful, when small pimples form round the mouth, and when the warmth, smell, and perspiration, sneezing, and the alvine evacuations are natural.

Should there occur, after the seventh day, sonorous breathing, listlessness and torpor, with thirst, constipation, hiccough, coughing, and vomiting with no appetite, the patient is in eminent danger. In such cases the person usually becomes very weak, and dies.

The most unfavourable prognostic symptoms of fever, when the patient should not be taken charge of by the physician, are when the senses are not in their natural state, or no longer act; when the person is weak, with sudden and severe attacks of fever; when the patient is decrepid, his extremities swell, and the fever remains during a greater part of the night; when affected with strabismus, and when his mouth remains open, and he is delirious. When he cannot be roused from his sleep, with the feeling of cold on the outside of the body, while he is hot inside, the patient is in great danger. In such cases the person generally dies.

Bátik-Jwara.—The treatment of this form of fever will depend on the stage at which it is examined. In the shivering fit, hot remedies are to be exhibited. According to *Sushruta* it is treated by enemas, the employment of errhines, composed of different medicines for removing the head-ache, and humours from the head, and by exhibiting the following infusion :

Cassia fistula...............(*A' bashwash.*)
Ruellea strepens..........(*Granthika.*)
Cyperus juncifoliao......(*Musta.*)
Black hellibore ....(*Tikta.*)
Myrobalan.................. *Haritakí.*)

Take 40 *ratis* of each, boil in one pint of water till a quarter remains, and strain. This quantity is for one dose, and is usually given in the morning and repeated for two days; various infusions of herbs, and barks of trees, are used in the same way. Prepared ghee with febrifuge medicines are used, when the above remedies do not cure the disease. In all cases the particular treatment will vary with the symptoms present.

The food to be taken in this fever is, first kidney beans (*Phaseolus mungo*) boiled, bruised, and eat with spice ; *conjee* with the juice of lemon, and warm water for drink. Long-pepper, hemidismus (*Sarura*), raisins (*kismis*), dill (*sataspispa*), (*ranuka*), of each 40 *ratis*, to a pint of water ; boiled down to a fourth, and taken twice a day.

Should this sort of fever be produced by severe exercise, or if the patient is very hungry, he may take broth with boiled rice, fish, *conjee*, and other such light food.

Should a strong evacuant medicine be given in the first stage of this, or any other fever, it will produce severe intermittent fevers.

Paittika Jwara.—This fever, like the last, has three stages. In the first stage give laxatives with cooling and bitter food. The *paltá* leaves (*Patolpatra*) 1 *tolá* ; with half a pint of simple water, or barley water boiled, and a little honey, for the taste, is given once a day, and is considered very cooling. The following cooling medicine is also given in this fever :—Take of

Parpataka, the bitter leaves of the Oldenlandea biflora,
Basaka...................(Justitia gaudcrussa,)

Katutiktá................(black helebore,)
Kirátatikta..............(Chiraita,)
Dhányaka.................(coriander seed,)
Priyangu.................(Panicum italicum,)

15 *ratìs* of each, or one *sicca* weight. A *tolá* to be infused in a pint of water until it is reduced to ¼, which is to be taken twice daily.

There are various other bitter remedies, all of which are said to cure this fever. It is also treated by covering the forehead with several cooling medicines mixed with water. When pain in the head is severe, with great heat, the person is recommended to sleep on lily, nim, and plantain leaves, to cool the body. They also recommend free ventilation, and residing in a cool situation. The house may be sprinkled with sandal—wood, and water. By a purgative you may prevent the recurrence of the disease, when only the preliminary symptoms are present.

In this fever the diet should consist of fried gram, or peas boiled in water, and strained. This is mixed with sugar and honey : the juice of acid fruits is also given.

Shlaishmik-Jwara, or Kapha-Jwara.—For seven days the person should not eat his usual food in this fever ; but should live on prepared peas, and the like. The stomach in the first stage of this fever should be cleared by an emetic, which will often cut the fever short, but this remedy is not to be used when the patient is very weak : after the emetic the juice of the leaves of Vitex negundo (*Incha* or *Sindubára*) is to be administered, with the powder of long-pepper, Heating medicines of all kinds are also used in this fever, as the diet should be light as well as heating.

Báta-paittika Jwara.—To remove this form of fever take of

Shunthì..............dry ginger,
Gulancha.............(Minispermum glabrum,)
Muthá................(Cyperus rotundus,)
Chirátá..............(Chiraita,)
Shálpánì.............(Hedysarum gangeticum,)
Chákulyá.............(Hemionites cordifolia,)
Byákur...............(Solanum Jaquini,) a variety of prickly nightshade.
Kantikárì............(Solanum melongena,) prickly night shade,
Ganirì...............(Premna spinosa,)

18 *ratìs* each, mix in water, boil to ¼, and take twice a day.

Diet. The decoction of *mudga*, a sort of pea, and the juice of *ámlaka* is often used. When there is much heat in the body we may give a decoction of gram, with the juice of the fruit of pomegranate for diet.

Báta-shlaishmik Jwara.—The treatment consists in exhibiting the root of long-pepper, *chabya,* (Piper chavya or Orris root, *Roxb.*) and root of *chitraka*, (Plumbago zeylanica,) and dried ginger : 32 *ratìs* of each are put into a pint of water, and boiled down to one fourth. Take this twice a day. Heating medicines may also be used in this fever, as chiraita, dry-ginger, *gulancha*, (Minispermum glabrum,) *básaka*, (Justicia ganderussa,) long-pepper, *lashun*,(garlick,) and *sindubára*, (Vitex negunda,) 20 *ratìs* each. Boil in a pint of water, till reduced to one-fourth, and take this twice daily. When the pain in the joints is severe, the vapour bath may be used ; and should there be great dryness of the mouth. in order to increase this secretion take salt, the powder of black-pepper, and the juice of lemons.

Diet. Boil in water the following medicines :—the bark of

Bilwa..........................(Ægle marmelos,)
Shonáka......................(Bignonia indica,)
Gambhàrì......................(Gmelina arborea,)
Pátalá..........................(Bignonia suave-olens,) and
Ganikáriká..................(Premna spinosa :)

of each 32 *ratìs*, mix in two seers of water, and reduce it to one seer. This is again boiled with some rice, and when cool strained.

Pitta-shlaishmik Jwara.—Abstinence in eating and drinking is to be enjoined ; the medicines that cure the diseases of bile and phlegm are to be given, such as

Gulancha.........................(Minispermum glabrum,)
Nimba............................neem bark,
Dhanyáka.......................coriander,
Chandana........................red sandal-wood,
Caturohinì.......................helebore,

ratìs 32 each, boil in a pint of water, till reduced to one-fourth; take this dose twice a day.

Perspiration is also to be encouraged, as phlegm shuts up the perspirable pores, and restores the internal heat to its proper place ; and water promotes the movements of the body, and cures the fever. Hot sand in a bag may be applied to the body, and by changing continually its position, it soon produces perspiration.

Long-pepper with its stem, dry-ginger, each 23 *ratis*, mixed and boiled together may be given twice daily.

Mixed fever.—In this fever the patient must abstain from food; he must be put into a sand-bath, and errhines, emetics, and expectorates administered to him. Should the person be drowsy several colyria are recommended. During this fever he should drink boiled water, which has been cooled.

Accidental fever, (A'gantuka).—Making offerings of fire, &c., to *bráhmans* will cure this species of fever. When produced by a bad conjunction of planets, gifts will cure it. By giving shelter to the traveller, setting him in a clean place, washing his feet, giving him food, will prevent the consequence. Another form of cure is going to the principal sacred temples, and making offerings through the *bráhmans.*

When it is produced by the passion of love there is no memory, the person dozes, is lazy, and delirious. In this variety every thing cooling is to be given; if *cough* is deranged, bitter things are to be given; if *air*, cooling things; if *bile*, sweet things. This fever is cured, when produced by poison, by the usual antidotes. When produced by grief, remedies for curing bile are to be used; when from lust, the person is to be comforted, and his purpose promised. If from fear, causes producing joy will perform a cure. When produced by an evil spirit, proper prayers will cure it.

Intermittent fevers (Bishama-Jwara).—At the time of the accession of the fever the paroxysm may be prevented by frightening the patient, by brandishing a naked sword before him, by advancing poisonous snakes near him, with the poisoned fangs removed, by the approach of dangerous elephants, and by the alarm of thieves. For a like purpose on the day of the return of the fever, emetics, purgatives, diaphoretics, or strong liquors are to be exhibited. These are to be given before the paroxysm is expected.

Anyejyuka. In this form use the following medicine:

Take of bark of the *nimba* tree,
Patolapatra,
Drákshyá,
A'mlaka,
Bibhitaka,
Haritaki
The flowers of the *mutá,*
Kurchi bark

two *máshás* of each, add a pint of water, and reduce the mixture to a half by boiling. Several medicines are also recommended to be mixed, and the steam from the mixture is allowed to come in contact with the body, which has been covered, so as to be exposed to the vapours.

Cháturthaka Biparjyaya.—Errhines are used for the cure of this fever. Certain roots are used for the same purpose, gathered on the nights of lucky days, and are sometimes tied to the hair of the head, and other parts of the body.

A'haka-jwara (*Nakra or Násá-jwara.*)—It is treated by us by abstracting a little blood from the nose by the point of a needle, or by rubbing a little rough grass over the diseased part. Errhines are also of use, and those who take snuff daily are free from the disease.

TREATMENT OF DYSENTERY, (*Atìsár.*)

In the acute form the person should abstain from food, and very light medicines should be administered to improve the dejections. If there is much pain and flatulency, he should take an emetic of salt, long-pepper, and hot water. After vomiting, very light food, of a farinaceous kind, is to be given. The physician should be careful in the acute stage not to stop the stools by astringents, or the like, as it will produce *Gulma*, anasarca, dyspepsia, piles, and drum-belly. When the stools are frequent, and very scanty, he may take myrobalan (*haritakì*). If the watery stools are copious, emetics, and the following medicines are to be administered. Take equal parts of

Haritakì......................(Myrobalan,)
Atibisa........................(Atis or Batula,)
Hingu.........................(Asafœtida,)
Soubor chullon............(rock-salt,)
Bacha..........................(Orris root, Acorus calamus,)

powder, mix, and give half a *tolá* or more, according to the age of the patient, for a dose, with a little hot water, wine, or *conjee.*

When deranged bile produces this disease, heating and stimulating medicines are not to be given; but he should take *conjee*, and agreeable bitter medicines. After some days of fasting, when he has some appetite, such bitters as

Atis..............................(turmerick,)
Atìbisha.......................(a plant *Aknudhi*, B.)

Indrajab..................(the seed of Wrightea antidysenterica,)
Pata......................
Rasánjana..............(Sulphurate of antimony,)

are to be formed into a decoction, and given two or three times a day with honey. In cases of bloody flux, boiled rice is given for food without water. In this manner the acrimony of the disease is supposed to be absorbed by the dry rice.

When the symptoms yield to these remedies; the urine increases, and is discharged without the passage of fæces, which are discharged freely and without pain, the appetite is restored, and when there is no uneasiness in the abdomen the person will recover. When there is swelling of the hands, feet, and joints, without any secretion of urine, and the dejections are very hot, the disease is considered to be increasing in violence.

In the chronic state (*Pákátisár*), when the stools are frequent, astringent medicines are to be given as follows. Take of

Sámangá.................(Lycopodium imbricatum, a sensative plant,)
Datakipuspa............(the flowers of Grislea tomentosa,)
Manjistá.................(Madar,)
Lodra......................(Symplocus racemosa,)
Mustaka...................(Cyperus rotundus,)
Sálmulìbesta.............(a kind of kino,)
Rodhra.....................(a tree called *Lodh*,)
Darimata.................(bark or shell of the pomegranate fruit,)

mix equal parts of these medicines in powder, and give half a *tolá* two or three times a day. When there is much pain, with costiveness, and blood is passed with mucus, take milk boiled with three pints with oily purgatives, and enemas of demulcent medicines with nourishing broths.

TREATMENT OF DIARRHŒA, (*Grihinì*.)

The bowels are first to be cleaned by an aperient stomachic; astringent remedies are then to be taken, with wine in the morning, and butter-milk. Asafœtida, and other stomachic remedies, as ginger, are useful. The fever and other diseases which sometimes accompany it, are to be treated in the usual manner.

The treatment of *Sangraha Grihinì* is the same as that of *Grihinì*; consisting of laxatives, stomachics, and astringent, light, and farinaceous diet.

TREATMENT OF ARSA, (*Piles*).

There are four indications for the cure of piles. The first is by medicine, the second by the application of caustics, the third by the application of the actual cautery, and the fourth, by the knife. When the disease is recent, and it is not accompanied with any bad symptoms, they may be cured by medicine. When soft and elevated with a thick base, they are to be cured by the use of caustic. When hard, rough, and large, by the actual cautery; and when the base is narrow and they are elevated and moist, they are to be removed by the knife.

The caustics are to be applied in the following manner: the patient is first to take some oleaginous and bland diet, such as rice and milk; the parts are then to be well fomented, and on a cool day, when there are no clouds in the sky, the patient is to be placed upon a table with a good light thrown upon the part. He is to be supported by two assistants holding his head and shoulders; and his loins are to be elevated with a soft cushion. The knees and legs are to be raised, and separated by a bandage passing round the knees, feet, and neck. The body is thus firmly fixed, and a little ghee rubbed upon the part. The patient is next to press downwards, so as to press out the anus. The piles are then to be dried with a piece of cloth, and the caustic fluid applied over the part by a broad pointed probe. The caustic is allowed to remain as long as is required to pronounce one hundred words, when it is to be rubbed off, and it is only when necessary, that it is to be again applied. When the piles become black, and are diminished in size by the caustic, the necessary effect has been produced. The part is then to be washed with a spirituous cooling application, whey, or water mixed with the juice of acid fruits. Dry the part, and then apply ghee mixed with the decoction of liquorice. A warm bath is then to be given, and pour tepid water over the body. He is then to be left in a room shut up, and is to live on a spare diet. When any other piles appear or when there are many, the application of the caustic is to be made every seventh day until the cure is completed. The applications are first to be made to the piles of the right side, then the left, and after that the part behind and before.

If the caustic is too freely applied the anus is destroyed, with burning fever, fainting, and discharge of blood.

When the piles are large and the person strong, they are to be removed with the knife, and the actual cautery applied. The diet is the same as after the application of cauteries. When the piles are not visible internal remedies must be used, such as myrobalan with jagry every morning. A hundred seeds of the *Myrobalan* are to be boiled in the hot urine of cows. Take them out after they have been boiled for some time, dry them, and then reduce them to powder. Such doses are to be taken as will operate on the bowels. The farina of the *Satabim* root is to be taken daily with milk. Tonic and bitter tinctures may also be used with advantage.

When the piles are painful use fomentations and poultices, with purgatives, emetics, and clysters. He should also avoid stopping the calls of nature; should avoid connexion with women, horse riding, &c.

TREATMENT OF AJIRNA, (Indigestion) AND DYSPEPSIA, (Agni Mándya.)

As indigestion, dyspepsia, and costiveness, are considered as only varieties of the same disease, the same plan of cure is to be followed in these cases.

In dyspepsia, myrobalan, dry-ginger, and sugar are to be taken internally; rock-salt and myrobalan; dry-ginger with sugar; the powder of long-pepper and myrobalan, or the juice of the pomegranate. In the morning, to clear the bowels the patient should take the following mixture: mix equal parts of

Dry-ginger,
Black and long-pepper.
The seeds of *Danti*, (Croton polyandrum,) the
Root of *Tribrit*, (Convolvulus turpethum,) and the
Root of *Chitra*, (Plumbago root, *rizia*,)

and take with a little sugar. This powder produces appetite and cures costiveness, pain (*sùl*), enlargement of the spleen and Jaundice.

In indigestion the following mixture is recommended: Take of Asafœtida, black-pepper, long-pepper, and dry-ginger, equal parts; make this into a paste with water, and rub it over the abdomen (*Charaka*). The decoction of coriander seed and ginger is recommended, as also a mixture of powdered myrobalan, long-pepper, and rock-salt in whey.

In the variety of this disease which is named *Ama-jirna* emetics are given, such as a decoction of *Bacha*, Orris root (Acorus calamus), rock-salt, each half a *tolá* in hot water. This will be repeated four or five times until the person vomits : or he may take as a diuretic the infusion of coriander seeds with a little ginger.

Bidagdha-jirna. Fasting is also recommended, and cold water to drink (*Sushruta*).

In *Bistabdha-jirna* warm applications are to be made externally to the abdomen. In other cases of dyspepsia take of

Black-pepper,
Long-pepper,
Ginger,
Ajamodá. (Ligusticum ajwaen,)
Rock-salt,
Jirait, (Cumin seed,)
Krishna-jiraka, (Nigella Indica or Sativa,) and
Hingu, (Asafœtida,)

of each equal parts. Mix and reduce them to powder; dose two scruples. Small quantities of wine and honey mixed with water may also be administered.

In dyspepsia, should the patient have sour eructations, with heart-burn, dried grapes (*kismis*) with myrobalan and honey, are to be given in the form of an electuary.

In *Bhasmágni* (*Bulimia*) the treatment should consist in taking purgatives frequently followed by heavy, indigestable, and oily food ; unleavened cakes of rice, ghee, and sugar ; the flesh of amphibious animals, as the buffalo, tortoise, &c. Fish is also recommended, mutton prepared with cocoanuts, &c., barley with wax-flower and water, ghee and sugar ; oily fruits, as walnuts, almonds, &c., so as to weaken the digestive powers which will cure the disease.

TREATMENT OF BISUCHIKA, (Cholera.)

The treatment of drum-belly, constipation and cholera are nearly the same. In all it is to be commenced by exhibiting a strong emetic. In cholera it is recommended to apply the actual cautery to the inner side of each ankle joint ; and hot external applications to the body. In all these cases fasting is enjoined, and after the emetics, medicines for correcting and soothing the pain in the stomach are to be used, followed by purgatives. When the faintness and purging has ceased, light easily digested food is to be given when hungry ; such as conjee mixed with stomachics, &c., clysters, with purgatives, such as a decoction of *Zowhori* (Convolvulus turpethum), castor oil, &c.

For internal exhibition, *Sushruta* recommends the following: Take of

Myrobalan,
Bacha............(Orris root.)
Hingu............(Asafœtida,)
Indrajab.........(Wrightea antidysenterica seed,)
Gringha......(small variety of garlic of a red colour,)
Sabardala......(rock-salt,) and
Atibisha.........(Atis or Bitula.)

The powder of these is to be mixed with warm water for use. Mustard seed with sugar is likewise recommended, also *Burhok* or *Bitlaban*, or black-salt.

Saindhaba......(rock-salt,)
Hingu............(Asafœtida,) with acid fruits.

These are to be mixed in water and taken two or three times a day.

The treatment of cholera must vary, and hence it is that so many different plans of treatment are recommended according to the prominent symptoms that are present.

Vomiting is to be produced by a decoction of *Bacha* and salt. When there is much vomiting it is to be stopped by the following preparation: Take 32 *ratis* of each of the following medicines:—

Caranja........ Galedupa arborea,)
Nimba...........(Melia azadirachta,)
Gluchi...........(Minespermum glabrum,)
Arjuna..........(Pentaptera Arjuna,)
Bacha.............(Orris root.)

Mix them with one pint of water; boil to a quarter. This will check the vomiting. For cramps, take mustard oil, rock-salt, and *Kusta*, (Costus speciosus.) Mix when warm, and rub it into the parts effected.

TREATMENT OF WORMS, (Krimi.)

For removing external worms, live mercury is to be rubbed with sulphur until a homogeneous black mass is produced; or the sulphurate of mercury which is to be mixed with the juice of *Datura Stramonium*, and rubbed over the part. In the present day a weak infusion of tobacco is often used.

There are twenty varieties of worms, each of which has a particular name. Their names are, *Juka, Antrada, Udarábesta, Khidayada, Mahágada, Chara, Durbakusama, Sugandha, Kaysida, Romabidhansa, Romadipa, Arambara, Saurasa, Matri, Parisajya, Kakìraka, Makìraka, Sausuráda, Sasulákiya* and *Sailiká*.

The thirteen first kinds of internal worms are curable, but the seven last are very difficult, or are incurable. The treatment in this case is to commence with the administration of an emetic prepared with ghee and *Sarasádi*, which is a mixture formed of various stimulants and bitter remedies. Strong cathartics are then to be given with clysters. The oil of *Biranga*, made of vermifuge seeds, is to be given with salt, and with the decoction of *Biranga*. The patient should at the same time be careful to avoid such food, and other causes which promote the generation of worms. He should take of the juice or paste of the *Palása* seeds (Butea frondosa), with the decoction of the *Balanga* seeds. The juice of the leaves of *Paribadraka* (Erythrina fulgens), with honey; or the juice of the leaves of *Patura* (Salincha B.) or the powder of *Biranga* with honey. *Biranga* powder should be mixed with the bread and used by the patient. Different preparations of iron, or the powdered root of long pepper taken with goat's urine are of use. Tin is recommended to be rubbed upon a rough stone, and the small particles thus removed from the mass is taken in whey. The treatment in cases of insects at the roots of the hair, causing them to fall of, is the same as that for baldness. The worms in the blood are to be treated, as for Leprosy.

Patients with worms should live on food mixed with pungent and bitter food, while the following articles of food are avoided. Milk, flesh, ghee, curdled milk, vegetables with leaves, acids, sweetmeats, and cold articles of food.

TREATMENT OF JAUNDICE, (*Pándu.*)

The *treatment* of Jaundice should be commenced by exhibiting several doses of mild purgatives, and emetics. The purgatives usually consist of Cassia fistula, or myrobalan with sugar. Before taking these he is to eat freely of ghee, which has been boiled in turmeric. The patient's body should be anointed with oil, after he has taken the above mixture for several days, and it has acted freely ;. the next object is to discharge impurities from the head by means of errhines with glysters : such as the powder of the oxide of iron, with ginger, black and long-pepper, with *biranga*. It is also recommended to give the fœces of the goat, mixed with black-salt *(bitlavan)*, and turmeric. These are made into a powder with honey, and taken frequently, for several days. A quarter or half a *tolá* of the powder of the bark of Convolvulus turpethum *(teuri)* may also be exhibited in sugar, as a purgative. A wine produced by fermented sugar is also to be used in this disease. Butter-milk and rice must be taken for a long time, as they will improve the appetite, and cure the disease. The patient should also take broths prepared with venison and prunes.

If air, bile, and phlegm are much deranged, medicines to cure these are to be given with the other remedies. If the patient, along with the above symptoms, has swelling of the anus, penis, and scrotum, and is senseless, with dysentery and fever, he is not to be treated.

In the form of Jaundice, called *kumbha káláma*, the rust of iron is recommended to be heated to a white heat, eight times, and each time it is to be thrown into the urine of the cow. This is then powdered, and taken with honey in doses of about half a dram.

In the variety of Jaundice called *Halimaka* prepared ghee with the juice of raisins, Minispermum glabrum (*gulancha*), and myrobalan (*ámlaki*), is often used with advantage.

TREATMENT OF HEMORRHAGIA, (*Raktapitta.*)

The hemorrhage from a stout person is not to be stopped at the beginning; as it otherwise will produce jaundice, dyspepsia, leprosy, enlargement of the spleen, fever, and *gulmah*. When the blood is evacuated from the urethra or anus, emetics are to be administered; and when from the mouth or nose, purgatives are to be used. If the person is very weak, the discharge of blood may be stopped by administering astringent articles.

When air, bile, and phlegm are much deranged, and the person strong, such a person should fast for some days, after which he is to drink conjee with a little rice, with sugar, lemon juice, and the juice of grapes.

Several decoctions and electuaries are recommended with preparations of ghee, to cure this complaint. The purgatives are to be mixed with the juice of grapes and liquorice root,—sugar, and the juice of other sweet fruits. Emetics are always to be used with honey, water, and the decoction of liquorice.

The diet should be cold water, and the flesh of wild animals, boiled rice, broths made of gram (*mung*), potatoes, and different other vegetables, seasoned with ghee, and mixed with the juice of the pomegranate, myrobalan, with the broth of pigeons, turtles, and shell-fish. Different preparations of rice as conjee with ghee may also be used.

The body should be anointed with cold oil, and cold applications are to be made to the body. In this disease the juice of the rose-apple leaves, or mangoe leaves, or *orgono* ; and the juice of the fruit of figs may be used with rice water, and the root of cucumber (*triposi*.) In other cases half a *tolá* of liquorice root in water ; the pulp of the seeds of *ingodah* with liquorice root, and sugar-cane bruised, are to be kept in a new earthen pot for one night steeped in cold water, with the flower of water-lily, and taken with honey.

If the blood proceeds from the nose he should snuff the powder of myrobalan. After a great loss of blood, the patient may drink the blood of animals with honey, or he may eat the flesh and unprepared liver of a goat with the bile. The juice of horse-dung with honey and sugar is also recommended. The powder of fried rice with honey, sugar, and the white concretion (*tobashia*) of the bamboo is also used. A decoction of the bark of rose-apple, mangoe, and *orgono* trees, are to be taken with honey ; and cold and sweet applications, both internally and externally are recommended.

TREATMENT OF PHTHISIS PULMONALIS, (*Consumption.*)

When the appetite is good, and the person is not very thin, and is careful, the physician may treat him. Ghee is to be taken internally, which had been prepared with *Stiran*, and other sweet, and nourishing medicines. This is to be followed by the use of mild purgatives, and emetics. Enemas are also to be given, and errhines to clean the head. The diet should consist of prepared barley, flour, rice, with animal broths ; when his appetite is good, give nourishing food, particularly the flesh of crows, owls, brahmany kites, rats, mongooses, wild-cats earth-worms, and all animals that burrow under the earth. These are to be boiled with oil, salt, and peas. The bodies of the animals are to be cut and bruised, and juice extracted. Wine made of grapes is to be given, with flesh of asses, mules, horses, camels, elephants, prepared in the usual way. The ghee of goats and sheep, with preparations of barley, are very proper. A mixture of ghee, honey, long-pepper, black-pepper, with *chubbo* (a pungent bulbous root), and *Biranga* (a vermifuge kind of seed), mixed with honey is also of use. The *Tubushin* (or salt of *balum.* or carbonate of allumina) is mixed with honey and *Til* oil. Another mixture is made by the powder of

Asuganda.........(Physalis flexuosa,)
Tila...................(Sesamum orientale,) and
Mása................(Phaseolus radiatus,)

with ghee of goats and honey. Garlic, pepper, &c., are given in gradually increased doses, and continued as alternative medicines. There are various mixtures recommended to nourish and give tone to the body, none of which it is necessary to enumerate.

It is recommended to eat the flesh, dejections, and blood, and live in the same house and in the same room with goats. The patient should carefully abstain from venery, avoid grief, anger, fatigue, and the other causes which produce the disease. He should also court the society of brahmans, physicians, gurus and study the sacred writings. This is recommended in consequence of the danger of the disease.

TREATMENT OF COUGH, (*Kása.*)

The *Treatment* of *Khyá Kása* is the same as that of *Jakháh.* The treatment of *Katazoa Kása* is as follows :—When the cough is produced by deranged air it is first to be treated by oleaginous medicines, such as prepared ghee, glysters, different animal broths, milk, and fruit. The patient may also take the decoction of

Shálparnì......(Hedysarum gangeticum,)
Prishniparnì,
Brihatì.........(Solanum melongena,) and
Kantikárì,......(Flacourtia sapida,)

with the powder of long-pepper.

Another electuary is prepared of powder of

Shunthi..........(Dry ginger,)
Shringì,
Kaná,
Long-pepper,
Barghul,
Jagry, with *Tila* oil.

When produced by bile give a purgative with sweet substances as—

Tiorì,
Tribrit.........(Convolvulus Turpethum,) and
Sugar.

He should likewise take a decoction of

Sarádì,
Panchamula,

with long-pepper and raisins. His food should be the broth of wild animals, good rice, and bitter vegetables. His drink should be prepared with

Bala..............(Sida cordifolia,)
Brihatì...... .....(Solanum melongena,)
Básaká............(Justicia ganderussa,) and
Drákshá............(Grapes.)

These are to be mixed with two seers of water, which are to be reduced by boiling to one: take this frequently. Milk with sugar is also recommended. When the disease is severe, and is produced by *phlegm* give first an emetic, with fried barley, and hot spices; such as long-pepper, saltpetre, and light and dry food, with stimulating medicines. For this purpose take a decoction of horseraddish,

Patkala,
Pushkara.........(Costus speciosus,)
Bhárgì,
Pipulì.............(long-pepper,) and
Súnthì..............(dry-ginger,) or the juice of fresh ginger with honey. Form these into a decoction, in the usual manner, and use it occasionally.

TREATMENT OF HICCUP, (*Hikka*.)

In the treatments prayers are first to the offered up to all the gods, on which occasion one nostril is shut up by the finger, and by the other nostril the air is taken into the lungs. Fear of all kinds cures it; and when a child is attacked if he be accused of having stolen something, or if he is threatened to be beaten, the sudden charge will cure the disease. Needles suddenly thurst into the skin, to produce a sudden surprise, will also cure it. Liquorice-root, mixed with honey, and taken in the nostrils as an errhine, or powdered long-pepper, with sugar and warm ghee, milk, and the juice of the sugar-cane will be of much use in curing the disease. If the person is not very weak give him a purgative and emetic; and use fumigations with gram, raisin, and other fragrant medicines. The ashes of the bones of animals, with honey, are also used for the same purpose ; or the ashes of the feathers of peacocks, with honey and ghee. Impure soda with lemon juice also cures hiccup, and hot barley water with ghee gives relief. A decoction of myrobalan is of much use, as also long-pepper, sugar, emblic myrobalan, and ginger with honey. The fried flesh of wild pigeons, and of different birds, porcupines, deer, granhas, formed into broths with acid fruits and ghee should be used. Purgatives, with salt or sugar, and clysters are also in some cases used with advantage.

TREATMENT OF ASTHMA, (*Swása.*)

In Asthma mild purgatives and emetics are to be given. Old ghee prepared with myrobalan, black-salt, and asafœtida, with powder of long-pepper. Ghee prepared with the five salts, as rock, black, common salt,

Sabaritulla, and
Sambari.

In other cases the ghee is to be prepared with the decoction o

Básaka............(Justicia ganderussa,)

or ghee prepared with Turmeric, Liquorice,

Sringì,
Madurikà.........(Anithum sowa,)
Byághrì..............(Solanum jacquini,)
Shunthì............(Dry-ginger,)
Rasànjana.........(Sulphurate of antimony,)
Banlochana, and
Mustaka.............(Cyperus rotundus.)

Acid fruits are recommended, with broths made of the flesh of birds which pick their food, as fowls, pigeons, &c. The heads of deer prepared with peas, and mixed with ghee are also used.

The following electuary is recommended. Take of the powder of the bark of

Byághrì...........(Solanum jacquini,)
Sringabira.........(Ginger,)
Sarkara.............(Sugar,)

The ashes of the quills of the porcupine, and the seeds of *Trikantaka*. These are to be mixed with the juice of the litter of the cow, honey, and the powder of long-pepper, and administered in the usual manner.

TREATMENT OF HOARSENESS, (*Swarabheda.*)

In treating this disease the body is first to be anointed with oil, and the bowels cleared by emetics, purgatives, and enemas. This is to be followed by the application of different kinds of errhines, gargles, and fumigations to the throat. When these remedies have been used without the desired effect the medicines recommended for asthma and cough are to be tried. When air is deranged, the patient should take ghee after dinner. The ghee is to be mixed with a decoction of

Kásamarda.........(Cassia or Senna esculenta,)
Bátaka,
Márkaba.

When bile is deranged, the ghee is to be prepared with the juice of

Arttagala,
Jabakshar...............(Saltpetre,)
Asmadá,
Ar,
Chritsak,
Amlaka...................(Emblic myrobalan.)

For diet he should use milk, rice, and molasses, with ghee.

When phlegm is deranged use rice, milk, and powdered liquorice-root with ghee; and other expectorant and heating substances, with cow's urine are also to be used.

The variety produced by fatness, is to be treated as in the form produced by diseased phlegm.

TREATMENT OF CHARDI, OR VOMITING.

All the varieties of vomiting are produced by disorders of the stomach, and in the treatment fasting is always to be enjoined. When vomiting is caused by indigestable matter in the stomach, emetics and purgatives are recommended. In all the varieties, light, dry and agreeable food should be exhibited. Different decoctions are also to be used according to the derangement of the humor as recommended in the treatment of fever. The juice of lemon, mixed with the powder of long-pepper and honey, may be sucked in the mouth with advantage in vomiting. A decoction of barley with honey, or fried rice boiled in water, and made into coujee is to be used. The paste of coriander seeds mixed with salt, and the juice of acid fruits will be of use. The pulp of prunes or myrobalan, with spices, will also be of use; as well as all articles possessed of agreeable smells. The broth of wild animals, bitter mixtures, and different kinds of agreeable food are all useful in checking vomiting.

During pregnancy the woman should be supplied with those articles of food which she wishes to eat, as the want of them will hurt the fetus, and will increase the tendency to sickness and vomiting.

TREATMENT OF SWOONING, (Mùrchhá.)

In general all the symptoms of swooning will disappear in a few minutes, with the exception of *sangnyása*, which requires immediate treatment. In all forms of swooning throw cold water upon the face and body, rub the body with the hand, allow a free circulation of air, and assist this by means of the *pankhá*. Wet the mouth with cold water, and approach sweet smelling substances to the nose. Such as the juice of sweet fruits, as of grapes, pomegranates, dates, (*khurma*,). the juice of wild animals, barley, and good rice; in like manner prepared ghee with a decoction of *myrobalan*; or a decoction of *Emblic myrobalan*; or a mixture of fried rice, grapes, honey, sugar, and the juice of the pomegranate, with the petals of the water-lily. The treatment followed in bilious fever is also recommended.

The treatment of *sangnyása* is difficult, and requires promptitude. Should the person not soon recover from the swoon, needles are to be thrust under the nails, and remedies which produce strong irritation, are to be applied, such as sweet music; and when the person is restored to sensibility, he is to have an emetic, and a purgative followed by the exhibition of *silájatu*. If these means do not succeed, the case is to be considered as hopeless. When the disease is produced by poisons, the person is to be treated as recommended under the head of poisons.

TREATMENT OF BURNING OF THE BODY, (Dáha.)

Take clarified old ghee and the flowers of barley, mix them well together, and rub it over the body. In old cases, water with vinegar should be applied to the body. Cloths wet in old and fermenting rice-water. In other cases sandal-wood reduced to a paste between two stones, with which the root of the Andropogon muricatum, a fragrant grass, is to be mixed and applied over the body.

The free use of the *Pankhá* is likewise recommended, and the patient should sleep or lie upon the leaves of the water-lily or plantain, and use the cold bath. He should take internally the juice of the sugar-cane, and different kinds of *sharbats*, the decoction of the stalk of the water-lily, a sort of fennel (Anethum panmorium), coriander seed, emblic myrobalan, and the fragrant wood of the *Padmakáshtha*, of each 32 ratis: boil in a pint of water so as to reduce it to half a pint, which is to be taken two or three times a day. Other antiphlogistic means are likewise recommended.

TREATMENT OF BURNING OF THE FEET. (*Páda-dáha.*)

In the treatment it is recommended that leeches should be applied to the feet, with the continued application of the mixture * of *masúra* (Ervum hirsutum). This is rubbed between two stones with water and applied to the feet. Butter is likewise recommended to be rubbed on the feet, which are then to be brought near the fire. With these means the usual treatment of *báta-rakta* (slight leprosy) is to be followed.

TREATMENT OF MADNESS, (*Unmáda.*)

The *treatment* of madness should consist of cleaning, and anointing the body with mustard oil: of eating ghee for some days, and then strong purgatives and emetics are to be given, with errhines, and mustard oil. Curious, or wonderful exhibitions are to be made before the patient; and he should be informed of the death of relatives, and friends. He should also be frightened by the alarm of robbers, by the approach of elephants and harmless serpents. The person should be beat with a whip, when he acts improperly; and he should live on light food, such as barley, and conjee water, made agreeable by the addition of carminatives. Ghee should be prepared, with a decoction of the following medicine: take of

Samap,
Elabáluka,
Elá,..................(Cardamoms,)
Chandana,
Debdáru,.........(Erythroxylon siduoxylloides,)
Haridra,.........(Turmeric,)
Kushtha,.........(Costus speciosus,)
Parminí,
Lariha,
Haranuka,

* Rather plaster, as it is thick, is spread over the part and allowed to remain.

Tribrit,............(Convolvulus turpethum,)
Dantì,
Bacha,
Tálìsa,.............(Corypha,)
Nabupisara.

These are to be prepared, in the usual way, with ghee and milk.

During the cure the person should be treated, as much as possible, with kindness and consideration.

When madness is produced by poison, the treatment is the same as that for poisons in general.

TREATMENT OF POSSESSED PERSONS, OR DEVIL-MADNESS (*Bhútonmada.*)

During the cure the patient should be treated kindly. A physician should commence the cure of a person possessed with a devil, by cleaning and anointing his body with mustard oil, he should be dressed in new clothes, and he should repeat the proper prayers, and act agreeably to the *shástras*; so as to satisfy the devil (*graha*) who is the cause of the madness. The usual red and white pigments are to be applied over the forehead, red clothing and garlands of red shoe-flower are to be worn, and honey, ghee, flesh, wine, milk, and articles of food are to be presented, for performing the *pùjá*. Some *graha* are satisfied with wine, some with goat's milk, &c., as stated in the *shástras*.

From the day of the invasion, find out when the devil will destroy the person, as each has a day particularly consecrated to him, and on that day use the proper means for removing the devil. The *pújá* is to be performed at the temple of one of the gods, by the physician, who if possible conveys there the person diseased; a fire is prepared, and flesh, &c., are thrown upon it, with suitable prayers. Some *kusa* grass (used for funerals) is to be sprinkled over the ground, a preparation of coloured ground rice, a cake of unleavened bread, ghee, and an umbrella is to be given to the devil. A mixture of sugar, milk, and rice boiled, is also to be presented.

When devils (*Asur*) afflict a person, the above remedies are to be administered in the square of the house. The removal of *Rákshyasa* devils is to be accomplished at the meeting of four roads, and in deep jungles. The *pújá* of *Pishácha* devils is to be performed in empty houses. When the devil has not been expelled by these means, with the prescribed prayers, other remedies are to be used. The smoke from leather, and hair, from the skin of a bear, or goat, from asafœtida, with goat's urine, are to be burnt, when even strong devils will be removed.

The other remedies are long-pepper, black-pepper, dry-ginger, rock-salt, asafœtida, myrobalan, and bacha, with the urine of goats, and the bile of fishes. These are to be used as errhines. Ghee and oil should be prepared, with the fæces, skin, hair, fat, urine, blood, bile and nails of the following animals: a lion, tiger, bear, cat, leopard, elephant, horse, and cow. These are to be mixed and used for anointing the body with, as errhines, or cold cream is to be mixed with these. Numerous other mixtures, of the same kind are also used in this disease.

Persons not liable to be afflicted by devils are, prophets, charitable persons, those who speak the truth, and those who attend to the orders of the *shástras*, and perform particular duties, and employ proper terms in addressing holy men. Those who have the eight qualities of the body, are always pure, humble, and wise, visit holy places, always govern their passions, and speak the truth; and those who pray, and attend to the prescribed ceremonies and are charitable, over such persons devils have no power. Devils only go about at night, and they live, under their eight chiefs, on blood, fat, flesh, and disgusting animals.

TREATMENT OF EPILEPSY, (*Apasmara or Mrighi.*)

When *air* is deranged, the treatment best adapted are enemas, the following decoction of *Jotela.*—Take equal parts of

Pamjamulì,
Haritakí, and
Goat's urine.

Prepare the decoction in the usual manner with ghee.

In treating this disease, when *bile* is deranged, the ghee should be prepared with the bile of

Goda,
Nokana,
Nága,
Pirsoto, and
Cow's urine.

This preparation is to be taken internally, and applied externally over the body.—The ghee may also be prepared in a decoction of

Tribrit,................(Convolvulus turpethum,)

Páthá,
Haridra,
Dár-haridra,..........(Zanthorrhizon,)
Anantamúl,...........(Periploca Indica,)
Pushkara,
Kataka,................(Strychnos potatorum,)
Bacha,...,...............(Acorus calamus,)
Sulence,
Biranga;

with cow's urine and milk, and some of its dung and curdled milk. This may be used for all kinds of epilepsy. Venesection is also recommended. Another remedy is, giving a wild boar purgatives for three days, then rice and milk; when this has been digested, he is to be destroyed, and the chyle in the vessels removed, and mixed with thin parts. It is to be put in a new pot, and when it has arrived at the vinous fermentation, it is to be given to the patient.

The general indications of cure are to give enemas in derangements of air, purgatives in bile, and emetics in the form produced by deranged phlegm.

In the form of epilepsy the body should be anointed with *átuk*, which is to be taken internally, and at the same time administer strong errhines, emetics, and púrgatives.

TREATMENT OF NERVOUS DISEASES, (*Báta Byádhì.*)

After distinguishing the disease, the next object is to find out the proper remedies for it, and how to exhibit them. When this is not attended to, the practitioner's reputation, and his income will be diminished; and if he does not use remedies on the discovery of the disease, it will be like a plant, which at first was easily removed, but when allowed to enlarge, and take deep root, it is removed with great difficulty. In nervous diseases oily enemas are to be used several times a day, and the body is to be frequently anointed with a mixture of

Kumkuma,............(Saffron,)
Agura,....................(Acquilaria agallocha,)
Kushtha,...............(Costus speciosus,)
Tagara,..................(Tabernæmontana coronaria,)

and other stimulants. Preparations of milk are also much used in this class of disease. The following mixture is often used. Take equal parts of *panchamula,* or *(bilwa), shonáka, gámbhári, pátalá,* and *ganikáriká,* form a decoction; or take with a decoction of Coriander seed, or *Kakalaidí*; a mixture of various vegetable stimulants and antispasmodic medicines; such as—

Kákolí ....(berry of the Calculus Indicus,)
Kshíra kákolí,......(resembles squill, and is often sold as such,)
Mudgaparní,........(Phaseolus Trilobus,)
Másaparní,..........(Glycine debilis,)
Chinrahá,............(Minispermum glabrum,)
Carkatashringí,.....(the root of the Momordica mixta, &c.)

When the joint is contracted mix together oil, ghee, the fat of animals, and the flesh of the crocodile, and turtle. Boil together for some time, and then let it be frequently applied warm to the parts. When there is much spasm, apply the mixture with a piece of cloth. Hot baths with hot douches, and shampooing are also of much use. Oily purgatives are useful, and hot oil in bladders is to be applied to the head, when there is head-ache. Emetics, and leeches to the part, are also recommended. Several aromatic, and anodyne substances with ghee are to be smoked or inhaled. Errhines of different kinds, made with prepared oil and ghee, are also used.

In this class of diseases the *diet* should consist of milk, with broth and meat, and sweet and acid fruits.

The person should wear warm woollen or cotton clothes, and the room should be in the centre of the house, cool, without any currents of air. The bed should be comfortable, and have soft cushions; and the person must avoid intemperance in eating and drinking, and intercourse with females.

When the *air* is deranged in the stomach, he should take equal parts (half a *tolá*) of the powder of

Chitraka........(the root of Plumbago zeylanica,)
Indrajaba,.....(seed of the wrightea antedysenterica,)
Pátá......... .. Cissampelos hexandra,)
Katuká,..........(Hellebore,)
Atibishá........(Atesor betula,) and
Abhayá,.........(Myrobalan.)

Repeat this medicine several times a day, and continue to take it for seven days. When deranged in the small intestines, oily purgatives, enemas, and food with salt are to be used.

When deranged in the bladder, diuretics should be given. When affecting the senses, prepared oil and ghee, are to be applied to the parts. When affecting the skin, flesh, and blood, venesection is recommended. When deranged in the large tendons, joints, and bones, pressure is to be used, as by shampooing and rubbing the part frequently with prepared oils, bandages, and the application of hot irons over the affected part.*

When the whole or half the body is affected, heat is applied in various ways to produce perspiration. The patient embraces hot stones, and is put into a hot room. In other cases dig a hole which will be heated, put leaves in it, and the person lies down in it, and when he is in a free perspiration he is removed to his bed. Venesection is recommended when the whole body is affected, and cupping is used in the variety which is local. When there is no feeling in the part; the application of the actual cautery, and of a mixture of oil, salt, and soot is recommended to be rubbed into the part.

The treatment of dislocation of the lower jaw consists in surrounding it with a cloth, and reducing the dislocation *(bapuskas)*. When the jaw is fixed by tetanus, apply prepared oil or ghee externally, so as to keep it well moist during the treatment, and then endeavour to open the mouth by force. When open a mixture of medicines to produce a free discharge of saliva is recommended; such a mixture is formed by the powder of long-pepper and ginger. At the same time the mouth should be frequently gargled with warm water. He should also eat garlic, with salt. Numerous other oils and medicines are likewise recommended in this dangerous class of diseases.

TREATMENT OF BATA RAKTA (A kind of Leprosy.)

The treatment of this disease is to be commenced by general and local bleeding; when the patient is not weak, or much reduced in flesh. Emetics and purgatives are then to be used. If the air is much deranged old ghee is to be administered, with the milk of goats, prepared with liquorice, honey, and sugar.

In other cases equal quantities of the following medicines are recommended.

* Rhumatism is a frequent disease among cows, and the actual cautery is freely applied with the best effects. Such cows are frequently to be seen marked all over the joints with these applications of the red hot iron.

Sunt,............(dry ginger,) mixed with
Singatuka,......(Trapa bispinosa,)
Kaserika,.......(Scirpus kysoor.)

In other cases a decoction prepared with milk and the five following medicines, is recommended.

Silparni,..........(Hedysarum gangetic,)
Prisniparni,......(Hemionites cordiflora,)
Kantikári........(Solanum jacquini,)
Bherhotí, .,.........(Solanum melongena,)
Kokurá,............(Ruellia longifolia,);

equal parts of these plants, are mixed together, to form the decoction. This mixture is called *panchamuli*, and may be used as follows. Take of

Panchamuli,.........and
Muhá panchamuli,..with liquorice,
Meshasringi,.........(Asclepias geminata,)
Sahala,...............(Pinus longifolia,)
Básaka,...............(Justicia ganderussa,)
Debdáru,.............(Ovaria longifolia,) and
Kantikári,...........(Solanum jacquini.)

These are to be mixed and formed into a decoction in the usual way. *Til* oil may also be prepared in the same way as the above. These mixtures are to be administered internally and applied externally. In other cases the powder of myrobalan with sugar is administered. A powder composed of five corns of long-pepper, is to be taken daily for ten days, and is to be decreased by degrees for a fortnight, during which time the patient should live on rice and milk.

The diet in this disease should consist of the simplest food in small quantities; as old rice, barley, flour, milk, broth of wild animals, and the decoction of a kind of pea (*mugh*). When the disease is violent, bleedings should be repeated several times, and emetics, purgatives, and enemas are to be given; such persons should live in a shut-up room, avoid currents of air, during the treatment; and he should sleep on a long comfortable bed, wtih soft pillows. The body should be shampooed, and he should avoid fatigue, sleeping during the day time, connexion with woman, anger, heating, salt, sour food.

TREATMENT OF DISEASES OF THE EXTREMITIES.

Give such medicines as decrease phlegm, but which do not increase bile. Avoid oleaginous applications, give emetics and purgatives, and apply hot applications to the part. Mustard and Coringo seeds, honey, and the earth of the white-ant's nests are to be mixed together, and applied to the part. Give at the same time *Silagita*, *Guguli*, long-pepper, and ginger. These are to be mixed with the urine of the cow. This form may be varied with the following. Take of castor-oil and *Guguli*, mix, and take internally : or a decoction of *Dasamula* with cow's urine, which may also be used.

TREATMENT OF ACUTE RHEUMATISM, (*Ámbát.*)

This should be commenced with fasting, diaphoretics, and bitters, tonics, and stomachics. Heating medicines with purgatives and enemas are also of much use in this disease. The sand-bath is also used, and on the leaves of the castor-oil plant hot sand is to be placed, and this is to be applied to the pained parts. The following vapour-bath is also recommended. Steep old rice in water until it ferments, the water is then poured off, and the following medicines are put into it:

The seeds of Dolichos biflorus, (*kulattha*,)
Teel seed, (*til*,)
The root of the castor-oil shrub,
Barley,
Linseed,
Boerhavia diffusa alater, (*punarnabá*.)

To four seers of water, take a *tolá* of each of these medicines ; boil, and in this state place the vessel with the mouth partly closed under the chair in which the patient sits, his whole person being covered with a thick cloth. Several pots are to be prepared in the above manner. He will thus remain for twenty minutes to half an hour.

Several kinds of plasters are likewise used. The following is a specimen of this class of medicines. Take of the roots of the

Abrus precatorius, (*Hingshirá*,)
Kebuka,
The Morunga. Guilandina sigrua,

to be mixed with cow's urine, and the earth of ant-hills so as to form a paste, which is to be applied hot to the affected part.

For purgatives take half a *tolá* of

Convolvulus turpethum, (*Teuri*,)
Sixteen ratis of rock salt,
And a little ginger,

with two ounces of conjee water. These are mixed and exhibited as a purgative.

Take of *dashamúla,*
Minispermum glabrum, (*Gulancha,*)
Castor-oil seeds,
Erundo and Mimosa octandra, (*rásná,*)
Ginger and Pinus debdaru, (*debdáru,*)

of each 32 ratis, mix in a pint of water, which is to be boiled down to a quarter of a pint. Take this twice a day for seven days. The tonic and stimulating decoction is prepared by mixing together the roots and seeds of long-pepper, the roots of Piper chavya (*chabya*). Plumbago, and dry ginger ; of each 32 ratis. They are to be put into a pint of water, and boiled down to a quarter of a pint. Take this twice a day. *

Diet. In this disease the *patola,* the fruit of the Trichosanthes dioica, old rice, barley, and a kind of pea (*mugh*), is also used, (*Charaka.*)

Sushruta recommends the patient to wear a warm dress, and to reside in a warm closed room.

TREATMENT OF SUL, COLIC, (*Gastroperiodynia.*)

Sul is diminished by the application of hot external medicines, frictions, or shampooing over the part with oleaginous applications, and drinking hot liquids. The pain in *air Sul* is first to be checked by hot applications, as bruised til-seed made into a poultice, and applied hot to the part, the external application of hot rice and milk is recommended, or flesh boiled, and applied hot to the pained part. For internal use take equal parts of powdered

Biranga,.........(A vermifuge seed like black-pepper,)
Sigri,..............(Silvius singio,)
Kampila,..........(A purgative root like rhubarb,)
Pateá,..............(Yellow myrobalan,)
Tribrit,.............(Convolvulus turpethum,)
Amblabitasa,......(Rumex vincarius,)
Surussah,.........(Ophiorrhiza mangos,)
Ashwakarna,......(Shorea robusta,)
Souborchsiloh,.....(An impure soda,)

one *tolá* is a dose, and may be taken with wine. This will at once relieve the pain. The following is another mixture. Take of

* *Charaka.*

Pritika,............(Nigella Indica,)
Ajjaghi,............(Cumin seed,)
Chobiká,............(Orris root, Piper chavya,)
Jawání,............(Ligusticum ajwaen,)
Marich,............(Black-pepper,)
Pipuli,............(Long-pepper,)
Sunti,............(Dry-ginger,)
Chitraka,............(Plumbago zeylanica,)

powder, and take it with warm water, wine, or hot conjee; or with the juice of the lemon, a decoction of prunes, or with asafœtida, or sugar.

The diet in this disease should be milk and oleaginous substances, and soup made of the flesh of wild birds, and of burrowing animals. Wine-whey is also of use with butter-milk, curdled-milk, black-salt, and vinegar, with diaphoretics and purgatives.

When the disease is produced by fasting the person may take hot milk, light rice puddings, or animal broths with ghee. When deranged bile produces this disease, mild vomits are to be used, and then drink cold water, and every thing cooling, while warm articles are avoided. Cooling things are to be applied to the pained part, as stone, silver, copper, or vessels filled with cold water. He should use purgatives and barley, rice, milk, ghee, the juice of the flesh of wild animals, birds and aqueous plants; and medicines that diminish bile, such as the juice of

Parasaka, an acid fruit, (Xylocarpus granatum,)
Mirdiká,.................(grapes,)
Kharjura.................(the fruit of Phœnix Sylvestris.)

The cure of *Sul* produced by phlegm is to commence by exhibiting an emetic so as to remove from the stomach what he has eaten. For this purpose, long-pepper, boiled in water may be used, and apply hot and dry remedies to the part. A hot regimen is to be followed; such as the use of long pepper, and dry-ginger, with the following mixture. Take equal parts of the root of the.

Gokra,..............(Ruellia longifolia,)
Maricha,...........(Black-pepper,)
Pipula,.............(Long-pepper,)
Sunti,...............(Dry-ginger,)
Bacha,...............(Orris root,)
Pátá.................(Aknuda, a plant.)

Katrahini.........(Black-hellebore,)
Chitraka............(Plumbago zeylanica,)

mix together in water, which is to be boiled until reduced to a quarter. This is given internally with nitre.

This last decoction will be found of great use in that kind of *Sul* which is produced by derangements of air, phlegm, and bile. It will cure it, as wind disperses clouds. In all forms of the disease castor oil, wine, whey, milk or lemon juice, will be of use. There are also different remedies, recommended according to the situation of the pain, whether it be in the scrobiculus cordis, bladder, or region of the heart.

When *Sul* is produced by indigestion, first use a vomit, enjoin total fasting, with such remedies as increase the internal heat or appetite. The other remedies used for *Gulma* may be given with advantage.

Sul may be cured when it is produced by either air, bile, or phlegm, being deranged singly. When two are diseased, with difficulty; but when all the three are deranged at the same time it is incurable. The treatment of the latter form is the same as above, varying the remedies according to the severity of the symptoms of air, bile and phlegm.

TREATMENT OF PARINAM SUL.

The treatment should consist of emetics followed by bitters, purgatives, and enemas. The following powders are also recommended. Take equal parts of

Biranga.........(vermifuge seed,)
Sunti.............(dry-ginger,)
Pipuli............(long-pepper,)
Maricha.........(black-pepper,)
Danti............(Croton polyandrum.)
Tribrit...........(Convolvulus turpethum.)
Chitraka.........(Plumbago zeylanica,)

make them into an electuary with sugar, and take it every morning with warm water.

Another remedy in this form of the diseases is

Sunti............(dried ginger,)
Tila..............(Til-seed,) and jagry, which is made into an electuary with milk.

Annadrabáka, is another form of *Sul*. This form is to be

treated with fasting, and the administration of emetics. A mixture of emblic myrobalan, yellow myrobalan, and ginger, with the mixture of iron (carbonate) is of use.

Another mixture is formed by mixing equal parts of

Biranga............(Vermifuge seed,)
Musta ....(Cyperus rotundus,)
Haritaki............(Myrobalan,)
Amlaki..............(Emblic myrobalan,)
Bibitaka.............(Beleric myrobalan,)
Gulancha...... .....(Menispermum glabrum,)
Danti...............(Croton polyandrum,)
Tribrit...............(Convolvulus turpethum,)
Sunti.................(dry-ginger,)
Pipuli...............(long-pepper,) and
Marich ....(black-pepper,)

These medicines are to be mixed with the powder of *Jawání*, (Ligusticum ajwaen,) and the carbonate of iron and water. The regimen in this form of the disease should consist of prepared rice in the form of conjee, and sugar and ghee with conjee.

Other *shástras* recommend promoting perspiration by hot baths, or vapour baths, by medicines to promote digestion, such as nitre, impure soda, and alum. It is also recommended to take eight *másá* of dried ginger, the root of the castor oil plant and barley, and mix them in a mortar with half a *seer* of water. This is boiled down to a quarter, and is to be tried as a dose; and it will generally relieve, or remove the pain of *Sul.*

TREATMENT OF RETENTION OF DISCHARGES, (*Udábarta.*)

When the *fæces* are confined, it is to be treated as for *Anaha.*

When *urine* is confined, *sabarchala*, (impure soda,) and other such salts, wine, cardamum seeds, with wine and milk, are to be given. The juice of the fruits of *ámlakì*, (emblic myrobalan) with water; or the juice of the sugar-cane, and the juice of the fæces of a horse or ass are recommended; as also the seeds of cucumber with water and salt, and other diuretics.

When *gaping* is checked, anoint the body with oil or ghee, previously heated.

When *tears* are confined, anoint the body with warm oil, a pigment of a hot nature is to be applied to the border of the eyes to make them discharge the tears; such as cloves rubbed up with honey and strong errhines, such as pungent smells will also be found useful.

When *sneezing* is confined, tickle the nose with something, so as to produce sneezing, and look at the sun so as to allow his rays to fall upon the mucous membrane of the nostrils.

When *belching* is confined a cheroot is to be formed of spices and ghee, which is to be smoked. Wine with soda, the juice of lemon and wine are likewise to be administered.

Should *vomiting* be impeded it produces leprosy &c. In such cases ghee is to be externally applied and internally administered, mixed with saltpetre or salt. Emetics should also be used.

When *semen* is confined, certain diuretics and decoctions with milk are to be administered, and the person is to approach his favourite wife.

When the *appetite* is not gratified, anoint the body with warm ghee and give it in the food, with hot drinks.

When the *thirst* is not gratified, the person should take resh conjee or barley water, with sugar and lemon juice.

When the *breathing* is difficult, rest and gruel are to be enjoined with animal broths.

When *sleep* is not gratified, give milk, employ soothing language, and what promotes sleep.

All kinds of *Udábarta* are to be treated as diseases of air, so as to open the closed up passages. and the body in such cases of disease should be anointed with oil and salt, and prepared ghee should be taken internally, enemas should also be used. If the disease is not cured by these medicines, hot applications are to be placed upon the abdomen, followed by oleaginous purgatives The person should take a decoction made of *Tribrit*, *Pilu*, *Jawini*, and the juices of acid fruits, mixed with water.

The following is also recommended. Take

Hingu,............(Asafœtida,)
Kusta............(Costus speciosus,)
Batsá,...........(Pothos officinalis,)
Sarjiká,.........(Impure soda,)
Biranga,.........(A vermifuge medicine,)

mix and form a decoction. These remedies will cure *Udábarta*, and pain. Suppositories will also promote the evacuations,

5.

glysters are also given, with the fumes of certain medicines. Other practitioners recommend, with the above plan of treatment, fasting, the hot bath, with purgatives, and hot carminatives.

TREATMENT OF GULMA, (*Swellings in the Abdomen.*)

When air is deranged the application of unctious substances to the surface of the body are to be used; but particularly over the tumour, after which oily purgatives are to be used, such as castor-oil, and oily clysters.

When bile produces *Gulma* unctious remedies are to be used externally, and he should take internally *Kákaládi* * prepared with ghee, followed by purgatives mixed with sugar.

When the bowels are constipated, milk with ginger is to be given; and the application to the abdomen of an earthen pot filled with warm water will be useful.

Phlegm. In this form, ghee prepared with a decoction of *Pipuládi*, a mixture composed of long-pepper, and other heating medicines. These are to be taken for some time internally, followed by strong purgatives and enemas. When air, bile, and phlegm, are diseased at the same time, the class of symptoms that appear most prominent will decide which of the above forms of treatment is to be preferred. When the disease is produced by retention of the menses, as sometimes occurs in women soon after delivery, eating improper food, or after abortion, or during the flow of the menses air is deranged, which prevents the flow of the menses, and produces *Gulma*. The symptoms of this form are the same as that produced by diseased bile, and at the same time the swelling moves about like a ball of clay, with the symptoms of pregnancy. When a round swelling is felt in the abdomen of a woman, the same as in utero-gestation, and it is so painful that the part cannot be touched, you are not to use remedies for the cure of this disease for ten months, and then you may prescribe medicines for it. The treatment of this variety is the same as that for derangements of the three humours in other parts of the body, combined with those for *Gulma* produced by bile with amenagoge medicines, such as potassa prepared from the *Palása* tree (Butea frondosa). This is to be mixed with ghee and taken internally, so as to separate and discharge the coagulated

* A medicinal mixture of an antibilious nature. It is principally composed of a medicine said to be brought from Nepal.

blood, which is supposed to be pent up, and produce the disease. Injections into the vagina of the female, with ghee prepared with long-pepper, black-pepper, and other hot medicines, are also recommended.

TREATMENT OF DISEASES OF THE HEART.

When produced by derangements of the *air*, the patient should first have his body anointed with oil, and he should take an oleaginous purgative followed by an emetic. He should next take the following mixture: Powdered long-pepper, cardamums, *Bacha*, asafœtida, saltpetre, rock-salt, dry ginger, and *Jawání*, with the juice of acid fruits and whey-wine or vinegar. He should eat good rice, with the broth of wild animals properly prepared, and occasionally use oleaginous glysters.

When *bile* is deranged the patient should be treated as in bilious fever, and all the decoctions and mixtures recommended in this disease are to be used. When produced by deranged *phlegm*, take an emetic with a decoction of *nim* leaves and *bacha*; with the mixture recommended above for derangements of the air. He should also take a purgative of *Tribrit* with ghee.

When produced by *worms*, the patient should eat meats prepared with ghee and rice, for three days; and then he should take purgatives of salt, and a decoction of aromatic plants. He should afterwards take wine with powdered *Biranga*. By this means the worms will come out of the heart. He should next eat *Biranga* powder (the best anthelmintic medicine), with barley for food.

TREATMENT OF STRANGURY, (Mútrakrichchhra) AND SUPPRESSION OF URINE, (Mutragháta.)

Different kinds of diuretics, alkalis, honey, wines, fomentations and injections, &c., are recommended in this disease.

The seeds of cucumbers bruised, and taken with salt and vinegar, or wine with salt, rum with animal flesh and honey, saffron with water and honey, different sharbats with acid fruits, especially pomegranate the fresh juice of the dung of asses with the decoction of *Abayá, Debdáru, Murba*, and *Madhuka*.

Cold water is to be given to drink with the juice of grapes, salt-petre, and other salts in water are to be used, and the body is to be anointed with oil, fomentations, and purgatives,

The *treatment* of *Sarajah*, *Asarí*, and *Sakará* will vary according to the humour particularly deranged. The medicines prescribed for stone are to be given in this disease, with a preparation of ghee, oil, and fat, with a decoction of

Shadanshtrà,
Asabiet.
Kumbhí,
Apushá,
Kantikárí,.........(Prickly nightshade,)
Balá..................(Sida cordifolia.)
Shatábarí,
Ràsná,...............(Mimosa octandra.)
Baruna..............(Capparis trifoliata,)
Girikarniká.

These are to be taken internally and used as glysters, and as injections into the urethra.

Another remedy to alleviate the pain is prepared by the juice of *Sadanstra* with jagry, and milk. A diuretic mixture called *Trinádu panchaka* made by the decoction of the root of sugar-cane, the roots of

Kusha ....(Species of grass,)
Kásha..........(Saccharum spontaneum,)
Shara,.........(Saccharum Sarah,) and
Ushara,........(Khuskhus.)

These are to be mixed with sugar and taken frequently.

When bile is deranged give purgatives, with the juice of sugar-cane, grapes, and milk. A decoction of *Sarasáda* or *Barnáda* prepared with oil. Barley water is to be given as drink.

When phlegm is much deranged, prepare oil with the above decoctions. When the three humours are deranged, the three kinds of medicines above stated are to be used conjointly as a mixture.

When produced by external injuries employ the usual treatment for such injuries.

In all these forms fomentations and warm bathing should be used.

TREATMENT OF URINARY CALCULI, (*Ashmarì.*)

When stone is threatened, ghee and other like substances are to be used, and will prevent its formation.

Stone is a dangerous disease, beinglike poison, or thunder. When recent it may be cured by medicines; but when of long standing an operation is required.

In the beginning give different decoctions and preparations of medicines, which dissolve the calculi; as *Pásánbheda. Basuka, Baskera, Ashmantaka Sotábarí, Shwadashtrá, Brihatí, Kantakárí, &c.* These decoctions are most useful when air is particularly diseased.

When bile is deranged, several different decoctions are to be used. The same is observed, when the calculi is produced by deranged phlegm. In all forms of this disease diuretics are to be used. If not cured by the above, an operation is to be performed, which is difficult and dangerous. It is consequently proper that the sanction of the Rájá be obtained to its performance.

The operation of *Lithotomy*.—The person should take ghee internally, for several days, with aperients. If very robust he should be reduced in strength. When the operation is to be performed; collect the necessary instruments, offer up prayers, and speak kindly and encouragingly to the patient. He is to sit on a table supported by a person behind, while his legs and arms are raised, and tied by proper bandages. The abdomen is to be well rubbed to make the stone descend. Two fingers of the left hand, well oiled, are to be introduced into the rectum, and the stone felt and brought down. Should the patient faint at this stage of the operation, it should not be proceeded in, as he will in this case die. An incision is then to be made on the left side of the perineum, a barley corn in breadth from the raphe, and carried down to the stone. The incision is to be larger in proportion to the size of the stone, and in other cases it may be made on the right side avoiding always the raphe. If there be more than one stone be careful to remove them all.

Care should be taken not to break the stone, nor to leave any fragments behind, as it will in such a case again form. These small pieces should be removed with a schoop called *Agrabakra.* During the operation the practitioner should carefully avoid the raphe, the seminal canals, the vessels of the spermatic cord, the anus, and the rectum. If the seminal canals, or the spermatic vessels are wounded, the person will become impotent. Wounds of the vagina and raphe, will produce much distressing pain.

In females the bladder is situated near the uterus, and care must therefore be taken not to thrust the knife directly forward, as it will wound the uterus, and the urine will pass through the vagina, forming a fistula.

The wounds of the bladder are always difficult to heal up.

After the stone has been removed, place the patient in a hip bath of warm water, to promote perspiration, and to prevent the accumulation of blood in the bladder. When this collection of blood takes place inject a decoction of *Kshirabriksha* (Ficus Indica) by means of a syringe. To heal the urinary passages; give sherbats, over the wound honey and ghee are to be rubbed; and remedies are to be exhibited to render the urine pure, such as barley with warm ghee twice a day for three days; after this time give sugar. rice, and milk in small quantities for ten days. Then take acid fruits, with the broth made of the flesh of game animals for ten days, and for ten more days promote perspiration by warm fomentations with oil and ghee. The wound is to be cleaned with the decoction of the *Kshirabriksha* tree, and other astringent medicines are to be mixed and placed in the wound. Oil and turmeric is also used with much benefit. If the wound does not heal up, and the urine does not pass by the natural passages, the actual cautery is to be applied. When the urine passes by the natural passages give sweet decoctions in the form of glysters.

When the calculi produced by semen cannot be dislodged from the urethra by pressure; an incision is to be made over them, and the calculi is to be removed by the assistance of a hook.

After the operation of Lythotomy connexion with women should be avoided for a year, as also riding on horse-back, on elephants, or in carriages; avoid at the same time swimming in water, or eating indigestable articles of food.

TREATMENT OF MORBID SECRETION OF URINE, (*Prameha.*)

The following are the names and medicines for the cure of diseased urine:—

1. *Udakameha.* For its cure use a decoction of *Párìjáta*, (Erythrina fulgens.)
2. *Ekhyumeha.* For its cure give a decoction of *Baijainti.*
3. *Sándrameha.* For its cure give the patient a decoction ot *Nimba.*
4. *Surámeha* is cured by a decoction of *Chitraka.*
5. *Pishtameha* is cured by a decoction of *Tamarinds.*

6. *Sukramehá.* For its cure give a decoction of *Durbá Saibala, Loba,* and *Kaseruka,* with other medicines of the like kind.

7. *Sikatámeha* is cured by giving a decoction of *Chitraka.*

8. *Swetameha.* For the cure give a decoction of *Trifalá,* formed by three varieties of myrobalan.

9. *Shanairmeha* is cured by a decoction of *Catechu.*

10. *Lálameha* is cured by means of astringent decoctions.

11. *Khármeha.* To cure this, use the decoction of the three varieties of myrobalan.

12. *Nilameha.* For the cure give a decoction of the bark of the banian tree.

13. *Kálameha.* For the cure use astringent decoctions, with honey.

14. *Haridrameha.* To cure this, use a decoction of *Cassia fistula.*

15. *Manjistameha.* To cure this, use a decoction of madder, and red sandal-wood.

16. *Raktameha.* Cure, use a decoction of *Gulancha, Casurga, Carjura,* and the seed of the *Tindaku.*

17. *Basámeha.* Cure, use a decoction of *Saptaparna* and also decoction of the bark of *Agnimanta* or *Sinsapa,* (a tree.)

18. For the cure of *Kandrameha,* use a decoction of the *Katiki,* and betel nuts.

19. In the cure of *Hastimeha* use a decoction made of *Tindika, Kapitta, Sirisa, Palàsa, Pátá, Murbà,* with honey. Another remedy is the ashes of the bones of elephants, horses, asses, and camels.

There are two kinds of *Prameha* ; one of which is congenital, and the other is produced by the use of bad food. In the first form give nourishing food, and in the second light food, with occasional fasting. In both forms the following articles are to be avoided, all kinds of wines, milk, especially curdled milk, oil, ghee, sugar, or sweet cakes, and acid drink. The flesh of domestic or amphibious animals are to be avoided, and the various kinds of fish. The patient is to use good old rice, barley, and flour, he should eat the different kinds of beans and peas, bitter and astringent vegetables, the flesh of wild animals without fat or ghee. The treatment should be oily purgatives, as castor-oil. This is to be followed by the exhibition of emetics. If there is much pain or scalding, give him antiphlogistic remedies, with the juice of emblic myrobalan, tamarinds, and honey. The physician should also exhibit tonics and astringents. He should drink sharbats containing honey, liquorice, and an acid fruit called *Kapitta*, with powdered black-pepper, and ashes of the dung of camels and asses. When the urine is increased much in quantity the patient should take prolonged exercise, as by walking and riding on horse-back, or on elephants. He should also drink different kinds of tinctures particularly those with preparations of iron.

TREATMENT OF SOMAROGA OR *Bahumutrá*.

The treatment consists in eating ripe plantains; in taking the fresh juice of emblic myrobalan mixed with honey, powdered *máskalái*, liquorice, *Bádám*, honey, ghee, and milk. The carbonate of iron and sulphurate of mercury is likewise recommended with honey; or the seeds of the wild fig with honey. Different other vegetable mixtures are also recommended with ghee in this disease.

TREATMENT OF GREAT FATNESS, (*Medah.*)

The powder of bitumen with cow's urine is exhibited in this disease. *Guguli* (Amyris agallochum) and the sulphurate of antimony is recommended internally, with honey and water, barley, *mugh* (a kind of pea), and other kinds of dry tonic food. Exercise, enemas, with tonics, and those medicines which make the body thin should be used.

TREATMENT OF ENLARGEMENT OF THE ABDOMEN (*Udara.*)

At the commencement of the disease the person should carefully avoid heavy food, or when not properly prepared, likewise oleaginous, dry, indigestable food and animal food, bathing, &c. He should live on barley, rice, and wheaten flour, or the like.

When diseased *air* produces this disease, the treatment should consist in taking preparations of ghee, laxatives with ghee, oleaginous enemas, and the abdomen should be rubbed with hot preparations; minced meat boiled and applied warm over the pained part is recommended; or rice and milk may be applied in the same way. He should also take milk with a decoction of *Bidárigandа*, and the broth made of wild animals.

Bile. Take prepared ghee, with a decoction of sweet medicinal plants, such as *Kákolì*, *Kirokákolì*, prepared ghee, with *Tawarhì*, (Myrobalan,) *Amlakì* (Emblic myrobalan,) and *Bibhìtaka*, as a purgative. Then take a decoction of *Botah*, and other astringent plants, with sugar, honey, and ghee. Boiled rice and milk, is to be applied to the abdominal region.

The treatment of *Phlegm(shleshmodara)* consists in administering ghee prepared with long-pepper, and other stimulant and carminative medicines. Enemas of cow's urine, oil, and a decoction of long and black-pepper and ginger, are to be exhibited. The abdomen should be rubbed with the following mixture: take equal parts of linseed, hemp seed, and mustard seeds with the seeds of *Mulaka* (horse-raddish). These are to be formed into a plaster, and applied with other hot medicines to the part.

The treatment of *Dakodara* is very difficult. The physician should, before commencing it, inform the friends that the disease is incurable; then he may try the effects of remedies. Administer strong purgatives repeatedly for a fortnight or a month. The root of *Aswamárika*, with *Jangá*, and *Kákádinì*, may be formed into a paste with wine, with which it is to be taken. Different forms of Nepal poison, as Aconitum, is said sometimes to be used. In other cases a sugar-cane is to be employed to irritate a poisonous snake, and when he has stung it, the sugar-cane is to be given to the patient to it.

The general treatment of the above forms of this disease varies with the cause. Should the derangement of air, and the accumulation of fæcal matter in the abdomen produce it, laxatives are to be freely used; such as castor oil, with cow's urine and milk or rice. These are to be exhibited for one or two months, without drinking water. The person must live entirely on camel's milk. He should take daily a dose of long-pepper, rock-salt, *ajwain*, with the oil of Croton (poliandas), milk, with the juice of fresh ginger, or myrobalan and sugar. The following medicine is also recommended. Take one thousand cloves of long-pepper, macerate it for seven days in the milk of Euphrobium. The seeds are then to be powdered, and to be taken occasionally. All forms of purgatives are useful in this disease, and many formulæ are recommended.

For treating *Plìhodara* (spleen) first give ghee, then promote perspiration by employing the steam bath, give rice with curdled milk for one day. General bleeding is then recommended by opening the veins at the bend of the left arm, and while the blood flows press the spleen, so as to evacuate the bad blood. He should then take nitre with asafœtida and rock-salt ; or a decoction of *Sabhánjana*, with long-pepper, rock-salt, *Chitraka*, the root of long-pepper, ginger, and nitre ; eight *tolá* of each ; add four seers of ghee, and four of milk ; and boil ; and when the watery part is dissipated, it is to be removed from the fire, strained and taken daily. Afterwards reduce to powder the long bivalve shells of the country by roasting them, and give the powder with milk. The liver is to be treated by opening the vein at the bend of the right arm, after ghee has been given, and perspiration has been promoted. The rest of the treatment is the same as in spleen and liver.

Baddaguda. In this disease it is recommended to give ghee internally, and rub it over the abdomen, while perspiration is produced by hot baths, &c. When the remedies are of no use, and the situation of the patient desperate, an operation is recommended, which is to be performed in the following manner: Below and on the left side of the umbiliacus, and four fingers breadth from the linea alba, an incision is to be made four fingers breadth in length, and the breadth of four fingers of the gut are to be drawn out, and the substance, whether stone or hair, or a bad secretion, which was the cause of the disease is to be removed ; ghee and honey is to be rubbed over the wound in the intestine, and it is then returned into the abdomen. Apply sutors, and treat the external wound as recommended in such cases. Avoid any currents of air after the operation, and carefully follow the physician's prescriptions. (*Sushruta.*)

Parisrábyudara. It is to be treated as the last ; but generally incurable. Warm baths, and a milk diet are recommended.

Asitis, (*Jalodara*, or *Dakodara.*) In this disease the abdomen is to be anointed with oil prepared with medicines to cure diseased air. A friend is to hold the patient in a reclining posture by the arm-pits. The practitioner then introduces a trocar an inch (four fingers breadth) below, and on the left side of the umbiliacus. The trocar is removed, and a tube is put in its place. The morbid fluid for 16 days is to be allowed slowly to evacuate itself; and a tight bandage is to be placed round the abdomen after the operation, so that the air may not swell the abdomen; this bandage must be continued for a considerable time. For six months after this operation milk is to be freely used with rice, or the broths of wild animals, with rice; and after three months and a half the quantity of water and milk with rice may be taken; and other three months light and wholesome food. The disease will be cured in one year.

TREATMENT OF SWELLINGS (Shotha.)

In this disease sour and salt food are to be avoided; curdled milk jagry, fat, milk, wine, oil, ghee, unleavened bread, and all indigestable kinds of food are to be avoided; the person should also avoid sleeping during the day, as also broths made of the flesh of domestic animals, and venery. When the deranged air produces this disease, medicines for curing air are to be exhibited; such as castor oil or the powder of the bark of the root of *Teurì* (Convolvulus turpethum). These purgatives are to be repeated at intervals for a fortnight, or a month.

When bile is deranged, ghee prepared with a decoction of astringent medicines, such as the bark of *nyagrodha* (Ficus Indica), and other such medicines are to be used. When phlegm is much deranged take prepared ghee in a decoction of the Cassia fistula, and medicines with the like qualities.

Besides the above remedies the following general indications of treatment are followed:—Different preparations of iron are used. In like manner equal quantities of marabuline and jagry are exhibited daily; or dry-ginger, black and long-pepper, with saltpetre, and the oxide of iron, in equal parts, are to be mixed with cow's urine, and are to be exhibited daily.

Diet. The diet is to consist of barley, with the decoction of *mudga* (a kind of pea), and flour; no salt nor ghee is to be used.

The warm bath, with a decoction of *nim* leaves, (Melia azadirachta,) *arka* (Calotropis gigantea), the leaves of hog-weed (*barshábhù*), is to be applied to the swelled parts.

Various kinds of external medicines are applied to dry up the swelling. Such as mustard powder, rock-salt, (Leea hirta) *singusta*. For the same reason strong purgatives and emetics are occasionally used. General bleeding is useful when the disease occurs without the presence of any other disease.

The juices of several roots mixed with recent cow-dung are recommended to be rubbed over the swelled part. In the same manner irritating substances are applied to the swelled part to disperse it.

In other cases milk is heated and the mouth of the pot with the hot milk is applied over the swelled part.

It is always proper to give oleaginous substances internally, to promote perspiration, and to rub the above mixtures externally over the part.

TREATMENT OF SHLIPADA, (*Elephantiasis.*)

When *air* is deranged in the part oleaginous substances are to be applied to the part to promote perspiration. Four fingers breadth above the ankle joint a vein is to be opened, and some blood is to be removed from the part. If the person be strong, give purgatives and enemas, which promote urine. Give castor-oil in cow's urine for a month, then take rice and milk, with the infusion of dry-ginger. The actual cautery may also be applied round the leg near its middle.

When *bile* produces the disease open a vein below the ankle joint, and use antiphlogistic and other medicines to cure diseased bile. The treatment followed in erysipelas should also be used.

In *phlegm* open a vein of the great toe, give astringent decoctions with honey, such as myrobalan with cow's urine; and rub the swelled part with a mixture of

Kotako,.............(Michelia Chumpaca,)
Amirta,.............(Minispermum glabrum,)
Biranga,............(Verbesina prostrata,)
Chitraka,...........(Plumbago zeylanica,)
Sunti,...............(dry-ginger,)
Dàri,.................(Laurus cinnamomum,)

mixed with the urine of a cow.

Give mustard oil internally, and use the juice of the clear *Patikaringo*. Impure potassa obtained from the ashes of the following drugs is likewise recommended; such as

Kákàdani,...............(Ficus oppositifolia,)
Kàkigungà,..............(Leea hirta,)
Birhutti,..................(Egg-plant,)
Kantikàriká..............(Ruellea longifolia,)
Kadamba pushpa,.......(a plant like *Kadamba*,)
Mundaru,..................(Asclepius gigantea,)
Lamba.......................(a bitter gourd,)
Sokonosà,..................(Cucumis sativus.)

This when taken internally cures elephantiasis and scrofulous tumours, and improves the appetite.

Fasting is to be enjoined for the cure of elephantiasis, and medicines are to be rubbed over the part; as *Dhaturá* root. castor-oil plant root, *Inchur* root, *Sajiná* bark, and mustard seed. Mix them with water. or *Sajiná* juice, and rub them over the part; which will cure even old cases. It thus appears that perspiration. the local discharge of blood, and purges, are the remedies recommended for this disease.

TREATMENT OF DISEASES OF THE MALE ORGANS OF GENERATION.

Diseases of the Scrotum (Briddhi).—With the exeption of hernia, this disease is to be treated as follows:—

In all these diseases riding on horse-back, sexual connexion, sedentary employment, and indigestable food are to be avoided. When produced by air, give the patient oleaginous food, and anoint his body. The parts are then to be fomented, and then give purgatives, especially castor-oil and milk. This treatment is to be continued for one month. The patient's diet should be broth made of wild animals, rice, and occasional glysters. If the swelling does not decrease by these means apply poultices, and when it suppurates evacuate the pus, taking care to avoid the raphe of the scrotum. The treatment is then to be the same as that of abscesses in general.

When the disease is caused by *bile*, and if it does not suppurate, it is to be treated, as other swellings produced by bile. If it suppurates evacuate the pus, and apply honey and ghee After this use such poultices as promote the healing action of the part.

When produced by blood apply leeches, give purgatives with honey and sugar; after which it is to be treated as swellings produced by *bile.*

When the disease is produced by diseased phlegm apply pressure with stimulants mixed with urine. If it suppurates, open it, and use such applications as will clear and heal the abscess.

In swellings when produced by *fat*, foment the part, and apply such poultices as will make the swelling be absorbed, such as *Sarosadi.*

This is to be mixed with urine, and applied hot to the part.

Surround the upper part of the scrotum with a bandage, and remove the lower and walled parts, taking care to preserve the testes and the raphe. Then apply a mixture of the sulphate of iron and rock salt to the wound, over which a bandage is to be applied. When the wound is clean apply prepared oil to heal it.

Mútrabriddhi (hydrocele).—Apply the same bandage as above recommended, then at the lower part of the side of the raphe a trocar is to be introduced. Leave the canula in the wound, and when the fluid is discharged, apply a tight bandage round the scrotum.

Antrabriddhi (Hernia) is incurable, unless when it is recent and situated in the groin, when it is to be treated in the same way as when the swelling is produced by air, that is by fomentations and oleaginous purgatives. When by these means the gut has been returned into the abdomen, the groin is to be cauterized (by a half moon cautery) over the part where the tumour was situated. In diseases of the scrotum it is also recommended that the skin of the right or left great toe be divided, according as the swelling is on the right or left side, and the wound is to be cauterized.

Brishanakachchhú, (itchiness of the scrotum (*pruzigo.*) The treatment consists in cleaning the part well, and applying simple ointment prepared with wax and bruised mustard seed, and *Satrak* (a small seed like aniseed); these are mixed, strained, and applied to the part.

TREATMENT OF SCROFULOUS SWELLINGS, (*Gandamálá.*)

When indolent and recent, follow the same treatment as of local inflammation, support his strength; ghee, fat and marrow, are to be prepared with a decoction of

Apehibati, and
Dasamula,

and applied to the part. Different fomentations, fumigations, and poultices are to be applied, and when they suppurate, open and discharge the matter; wash the wound with a decoction of

Bilwa,............(Ægle marmelos,)
Arka,...............(Calotropis gigantea,) and
Arjuna,............(Pentaptera arjuna.)

A poultice made of *Tila*, and the leaves of the castor-oil tree mixed with salt, and applied to the part. Then apply oil which has been prepared with a decoction of

Rásná............(Mimosa octandra,) and
Sarala,...........(Pinus longifolia.)

When the disease is produced by bile, apply leeches, with milk and water, and other cold applications. Aperients are likewise to be given, and a paste made of

Madhuka,...........(Bassia latifolia,)
Jambi, or
Juna, and
Betasa, with
Sugar.

When it suppurates open, and wash with a decoction of astringent barks. Then apply a poultice, and ghee prepared with liquorice, and other sweet medicines ; as

Kákolí,.........(Coclus Indicus,)
Kshárakákolí, &c.

When produced by *phlegm* use rubbing with the finger, or with iron, stone, or a piece of bamboo : make also a paste of

Bekantaká,
Arikbuda,
Gunja...............(Abrus precatorius,)
Kakádmi, and
Tapasabirka,

and apply to the part. If not situated in a vital part remove the tumour with the knife, and when the blood is stopped treat it as a simple wound.

Tumours of the Neck, (*Manskunder*,) is a variety of the *Gandamálá* or scrofulous swellings. They are hard and large, and when they suppurate they should be opened. After which the cavity is to be cleaned with astringent washes. Detergent medicines are also to be used, as honey, ghee, and caustic preparations Then apply oil prepared with a decoction of

Biranga,
Páthá,.........a plant called *Aknadi*, and
Rasaní,............(or turmeric.)

When the tumours are produced by fat apply a paste made of Sesamum seed. Then two folds of cloth are to be placed over the part, and a hot iron is to be applied frequently over the part. If the tumour is not removed in this way, the knife must be had recourse to. In this and in all scrofulous affections, emetics and purgatives are to be occasionally exhibited. Errhines are also of use. The actual cautery is to be applied across the arm immediately above the wrist leaving an interval of the breadth of a finger between each application.

TREATMENT OF GOITRE, (*Galaganda.*)

Foment the parts with steam, by means of a tube proceeding from a vessel, in which those vegetable remedies are boiling which cure diseased air. When air is deranged, the steam of warm milk is used; and warm poultices prepared with flesh and oil are to be applied, and an opening made into it, and it is then to be treated like a common inflammation. The following external applications are also recommended. The seeds of

Sana,
Atasí, ...(Linum usitatissinum,)
Múlaka,........(Raphanus sativus,)
Sigru,...........the pulp of the
Pilu, and
Tìla,.............Sesamun seed, are made into a poultice and applied to the swelling. A paste made with urine, and the juice of acid fruits, such as

Aquiseka,
Brikshaka,............(Wrightea antidysenterica,) and
Tilaka, are recommended.

Oil prepared with

Bala,............(Sida cordifolia,)
Shwetbalá,.....(Vallisneria octandra,) and
Pìtabalá; or with
Amartabalá,
Nimba,..........(Melia azadirachta,)
Hansiabia,
Trikaka,

and long-pepper; is used internally.

When produced by phlegm, fomentations are to be applied as above; open the swelling, and oil prepared with different salts, and with the ashes of long-pepper, and other heating medicines is to be exhibited internally. Use also externally, paste made of *gunja* with the water of the ashes of *palása,* and applied to the part hot.

Diet.—Use barley, a decoction of *mudga* with cow's urine, or with powdered long and black-pepper, ginger, and honey.

When caused by fat apply a paste made of

Simá,
Sudda,
Mandura,
Danti,...............(Croton polyandrum,) and
Rasánjana,.........(Sulphurate of antimony.)

The gum rosin of the *sál* tree, with cow's urine may be used daily: or make an incision, remove the fat, and sow up the wound; then apply ghee and honey to the part, or hot oil. The patient is to live on a preparation of barley, and apply a tight bandage to the part. The decoction of the three kinds of myrobalan is also recommended.

TREATMENT OF BHAGANDARA, (*Fistula-in-Ano.*)

When there is only a swelling, use antiphlogistic regimen, as scanty diet, purgatives, and fomentations to the part. Cold applications, and poultices to the part are of use in some cases. Give these decoctions to diminish the swelling; and if they are not sufficient to remove the disease, apply such medicines as promote suppuration. The swelling is then to be opened, and treated as in other swellings of the same kind. Emetics and purgatives will also be administered with advantage in this disease.

When the fistula is open, and there is an external and internal apperture, place the patient on a bed, introduce a director, and divide the flesh between the fistula and anus; then apply caustic or the actual cautery to the wound. When several fistulæ exist, perform the operation for one, and then for another. When they communicate with each other open them all, if external, so that they be all formed into one wound. But when they do not communicate with each other, the opening is to be made separately into the gut. After the operation the actual cautery is to be applied, by means of a red hot probe.

The form called *Satapanaka* is incurable in a weak and fearful person. When the person will not submit to an operation apply fomentations and poultices, and give him tonic medicines, and apply ghee, and oil to the part. By these means the fistulous opening may be healed up.

In *Utragraba* use a similar plan of treatment as in the last case, but the actual cautery is not required. Caustic in this case is sufficient; after which apply a poultice and bandage to the part. On the third day clean the part, and apply healing medicines.

In *Parisrába* the part is to be divided as in the other forms, and apply the actual or potential cautery to the part. After which warm oil is to be applied to the part, with fomentations and poultices; aperient medicines are likewise to be given.

When a fistula-in-ano either of the internal or external kind, occurs in children, neither caustic, cautery, nor the knife, are to be employed. In this case a small bougie is to be introduced. It is composed of *Arakboda*, turmeric, and *Kula*, mixed with ghee and honey. This is to be introduced into the fistulous opening, which will by this means heal up.

In the last or accidental form of fistula, first remove the bone, and the fistulous opening being enlarged in the usual way, the actual cautery is to be applied to its surface, and the means for removing worms are to be resorted to in this disease.

The after treatment of the wounds and ulcers should resemble those recommended under the head of surgery.

For one year after the cure the patient should avoid any great excitement, as horse exercise, fatigue, connection with women, anger, and heavy indigestable food, which might produce a relapse.

TREATMENT OF SORES ON THE GENITAL ORGANS, (*Upadangsha.*)

There are five different forms of these sores. These are *Bátika*, *Paittika*, *Shleshmika*, *Sannipátika*, *Ayantuka*, or *accidental injuries* of the organs of generation.

The treatment of the above local diseases of the genitals is as follows:

For the cure of *Bátika* apply ghee, or some oleaginous matter to the local disease, and give the same internally, to promote perspiration. Open a vein of the penis, or apply leeches to that organ, so as to remove any unhealthy humours that may be there; and for the same purpose administer strong purgatives and emetics. For the former medicine, glysters may be substituted when the patient is weak. The parts are next to be fomented, and then apply to them poultices of flour, mixed with the powder of the castor-oil seed.

Paittika. In this variety apply fomentations of milk and water, sugar and water, or honey and water. The following poultices are then to be applied:—Take of

Gairíka,.........(Yellow earth,)
Anjana,.........(Sulphate of antimony,)
Lukarna,
Sáribá,...........(Echites frutescens,)
Jashtimadhu,....(liquorice,)
Ushìra,
Kusha,............(Grass,)
Padmaka,.........(a fragrant wood,)
Sandal-wood and water-lily.

Mix these together with ghee and use it as a poultice.

Shleshmika, is produced by a diseased state of the phlegm in the part, and is treated by fomenting with a decoction made of the bark of

Sála,...................(Sal tree,)
Ashwakarna,.........(a kind of Sala tree,) and
Dhaba,.................(Grislea tomemtosa.)

The same barks may be mixed with wine and mustard oil, and used as a poultice.

By thus employing bleeding and other antiphlogistic means, according to the nature of the case; by the use of fomentations and poultices, with the assistance of emetics and purgatives, this disease will be most easily cured. Washing the sores with astringent decoctions, will also be found of much use. Much care is required in the treatment, when accompanied with sloughing or suppuration of the parts. In this case the abscess is to be immediately opened, as soon as it is discovered; and then apply *til*, honey, and *ghee*. A fomentation of the leaves of

Karabíra,........(Oleander,)
Játí,................(Jasmin,) and
Arakbada,.......(Cassia fistula,) is then to be applied

to the part. Various mixtures of powders are recommended to be applied with honey to these sores of the genitals. The following may be given as an example. Take of

Sourástra mirtiká,......(a kind of earth,)
Gaerika,
Tute,.........................(Sulphate of copper,)
Pushpaka..................(sulphate of zinc,)

Kasísa,......................(Sulphate of iron,)
Saindhaba,................(rock-salt.)

These, and other medicines of the same kind, with various astringent powders and decoctions, are used. When the disease is produced by a derangement of the three humours the treatment recommended for foul ulcers is to be followed. If the parts have sloughed, or gangrene has taken place, the dead part is to be separated, the actual cautery applied, and the part is to be dressed with honey and ghee.

In *Paribarttiká* (*Phymosis*) ghee is to be applied to the part with warm fomentations followed by poultices, which are to be continued for from three to five days. Ghee is again to be applied, and the skin is then to be pulled gently backwards. When in its natural position apply fomentations, administer oleaginous food, with animal broths, and ghee.

The same treatment is to be followed in Pariphymosis, only instead of backwards, pull the prepuce forward.

In *Niruddaprakasha* introduce a metalic, wooden, or gumelastic canula, after the parts have been rubbed with oil. Then the size of the canula is to be increased every third day, so as to increase the size of the passage of the urethra.

Should the prepuce adhere to the glans divide them, and heal the wound in the ordinary way.

In *Shúkadosha*, astringent decoctions and oils are to be used, after the application of leeches, fomentations, and poultices. When matter forms it is to be evacuated and the abscess cleaned with tonic decocticns. The ulcers are to be healed by the application of prepared oil.

When sloughing takes place it is to be treated, as when it occurs in other parts. In all these forms of disease the antiphlogistic treatment is to be employed, particularly purgatives, and the local application of astringent, and healing powders.

TREATMENT OF LEPROSY, (*Kushtha or Kuth.*)

Leprosy commences first in the skin, and gradually extends deeper and deeper affecting the different essential parts, as flesh, blood, fat, &c. Thus like the small shoots of the Banian tree, which are at first confined to the surface, they advance deeper and deeper, until they extend over the whole body. In the first stage, when it is superficial, the use of proper diet and medicines may cure it; but when it has extended to a greater distance, the difficulty of curing it becomes much greater.

Diet.—In leprosy, flesh, with the exception of that of wild animals, and oleaginous articles of food are not to be used; as also hard food, milk, curdled milk, certain kinds of pulse; sour articles or sweet, prepared from sugar-cane. Improper and indigestable articles of food, or eating too often of roasted or heating food are to be avoided, and also sleeping in the day time, and connexion with woman. Good and old rice is to be used with barley, flour, and peas (*mugh*) boiled in water, and mixed with the leaves of *nimba*. Such vegetables as contain a bitter principle are useful. In other cases, barley is recommended to be steeped in cow's urine for a night and then dried in the sun. This is to be repeated seven days; then fry it, and some of it is to be taken every morning with a decoction of the following bitters,

Kantikári,.........(Solanum Jacquini,) and
Nimba,.........(Melia Azadirachta, &c.)

Prepared oils are to be used to anoint the body with.

The ulcers are to be cleaned with astringent decoctions; with an oily preparation called Vajraka, and a paste or liniment of the aragbadha (Cassia fistula). The water with which the person washes or bathes should be impregnated with *khayar*, catechu, which also should be mixed with the drinking water.

In the beginning of the disease purgatives and emetics are first to be administered. If the leprosy is confined to the skin evacuant medicines, and smearing the body with different sorts of medicines are of use. If confined to the blood it is to be purified by evacuants, smearing the body with proper medicines, drinking bitter and astringent decoctions, and venesection. When confined to the flesh the remedies are the same as those of blood, with tonic tinctures, of various kinds. When confined to the fat it is incurable; but the progress of the disease may be checked by proper diet and medicines, especially tonics. When the bones are affected it is incurable, and should not be treated.

When marrow is diseased the man will soon die. In the seven severe forms of leprosy, besides emetics and purgatives, glysters, supposotories, with errhines are to be used. If these five forms of medicines have been employed without effect, the case may be considered as hopeless.

When *air* produces leprosy, prepared ghee, with astringent tonics are to be used; when *phlegm*, emetics; when *bile*, blood is to be removed from the person, and purgatives are to be administered.

The following mixtures are much recommended in leprosy. Take equal parts of

Meshashringí..........(Asclepias geminata, &c.)
Shwadangshtrá,......(Flacourtia catafracta,)
Gulancha...............(Minispermum glabrum,)
Shángashthá,..........(Leea hirta,)

mix with *Panchamuli*. This mixture consists of equal parts of the bark of

Bilwa,...............(Ægle marmelos,)
Sanáka,.............(Bignonia indica,)
Gámbhári..........(Gmelina arborea,)
Pátalá...............(Bignonia Suaveolens,) and
Ganikáriká,.........(Premna spinosa.)

These medicines are to be boiled in water, shaken, mixed with ghee, and boiled down till the watery part is dissipated. This to be taken internally, mixed with oil, and rubbed over the body. In other cases the ghee is prepared in the same way with

Bhallátaka,.........(Marking Nut,)
Abhayá,.............(Myrobalan,)

ana a vermifuge plant called *biranga*. It resembles black-pepper, is prepared as above, and used for the cure of all the different forms of leprosy.

Blood-letting is used frequently in the cure of leprosy, and is abstracted from different veins. When prominent patches form, scarifications, leeches or caustics, are to be used.

Various medicines are recommended for rubbing over the body. They are usually of a stimulating nature. The following is one of these. Take of

Haritála,............(Yellow arsenic,)
Manahshilá,.........(Red arsenic,)
the juice of the Madar, (*Arka*,)
a kind of horse-raddish called *Sigru* or *Shobhánjana*,
black-pepper, and the seed of Sesamum, (*Til*,)

mix together, in equal parts. These are to be rubbed with water, and applied to the surface affected. There are seven other varieties of such mixtures. The following is recommended. Take of the leaves of Cassia fistula *(sondál)*, and mix them with butter-milk, and rub it over the diseased part, particularly where there are tubercles. Others recommend the froth of the sea *(samudra-phena)*, after it has been dried, to be rubbed over the diseased parts.

The following may therefore be considered as the best means of curing leprosy. Use freely catechu by mixing it with the water of the patient's bath, in his drinks, food and medicine, while he avoids animal food, wine, and intercourse with women. When the disease is subdued, use purgatives freely to prevent a relapse.

With these means, certain diet, wearing clean clothing, and a proper degree of exercise is to be used. Such treatment will generally cure the disease: especially if emetics are given every fortnight, purgatives every month and venesection twice a year. Two tolás of the powder of turmeric in cow's urine are to be taken at the same time, every day for one month; and every third night an errhine is to be exhibited.

The following mixture is also much recommended. Take of the bark of the *nibma* tree, the leaves of a kind of cucumber commonly called Palwal, (*Paltá*,) the leaves of Solanum Jacquini, (*Kantikárì*,) Minispermum glabrum, (*Gulancha*,) with the bark of Justicia ganderussa, (*Básaka*,) of each ten *pols* (about ℥iv.) mix them with 64 seers of water; and boil to 16 seers. Remove it from the fire, and add four seers of ghee by degrees, and again put it on the fire until the water is dissipated. To this medicine add the

Harìtakì,............(Paste of Myrobalan,)
Bibhìtakì............(Terminalia belerica,) and
Amlakì,.............(Phylanthus emblica;)

of each two pols,* 5 tolás, and 2 másás, and 7 ratis, are to be added. The whole is to be mixed in a mortar, to which ghee is to be added; it is again to be placed over the fire for a short time, and when mixed, it is then to be strained through cloth. This, taken internally, is said to cure leprosy, the 80 diseases produced by deranged air, the 40 diseases of bile, and the 20 diseases of phlegm. It is also useful in bad boils, worms, piles, and the five kinds of cough. Other mixtures equally efficacious in curing numerous diseases, are recommended. These vaunted

* Eight tolás make one pol.

qualities of certain mixtures is to encourage the patient, as well as the practitioner ; and their inefficiency explains the numerous other mixtures which are recommended as substitutes.

Should worms form in leprous ulcers, a paste made of the bark of Nerium odorum (*Assamára*), and the seeds of a vermifuge plant called *biranga*, with cow's urine, is to be applied to the sore.

White Leprosy.—The diet in the white leprosy is the same as in the black.

The treatment of white leprosy consists in the exhibition of external, and internal medicines.

External Medicines.

Take of the flowers and leaves of

Pùtìka,............(Cæsalpinia bonducella,)
Akun,..............(Calotropis gigantea,)
Sthahì,.............(Euphorbium,)
Baruna,...........(Tapia cratæva,)

in equal proportions. Mix to the consistence of paste, with the urine of the cow, and apply to the part affected. The ashes of the skin of elephants and tigers ; and the powder of the flying bug (*pàdapoká*), is also used. Another remedy is the fæces of a fowl which has been kept fasting for three days ; during which time it is only to receive a mixture of the seed of Cassia tora (*prepunára*), and liquorice root. The fæces is to be rubbed over the part ; and repeat the application daily for a month, during which time the same mixture is occasionally to be given to the fowl. Another external application is prepared as follows: The juice of the mango tree is to be mixed with the bark and leaves of the murabuli, the mixture is to be put into a copper vessel, and mixed with the juice of the Ficus Indica (*bot tree*). It is then burnt, and the ashes are to be mixed with a decoction of myrobalan, and mustard oil. This medicine is to be rubbed over the affected part.

The *Internal Medicines* employed for white leprosy are very numerous. The following mixture may be taken as an example. Take of the powder of the root of Plumbago Zeylanica (*Chitrakah.*) black-pepper, dry-ginger, and long-pepper ; macerate them in cow's urine in an earthen water-pot, in which ghee had been kept, and some honey ; keep the mixture for a fortnight, strain, and give one tolá for a dose.

TREATMENT OF URTICARIA ? (*Sitapita.*)

In *Udordah*, mustard oil is to be rubbed over the body; in other cases turmeric, *dub* grass (Panicum dactylon), and the urine of the cow, are to be mixed and rubbed over the body. The warm bath is of great use; and a decoction of *nimba* leaves, as an emetic and purgative, with one tolá of *trifalá** and half a tolá of *teori* or Convolvulus turpethum and *tribrit*, or castor oil. If for several days the person takes the powder of myrobalan (*ámlaki*), liquorice root with sugar; or Legusticum ajwaen (*jawáni*) and sugar, and uses the proper diet, he will be cured of the disease. The juice of fresh ginger, with old impure sugar, is also used. In *Sitapita*, the same treatment is to be employed; in *Khata*, tonic medicines are to be given with blood letting. The powder of the *nimba* leaves, and emblic myrobalan (*ámlaki*), are to be taken internally. He should also take rice prepared with horse raddish, and the gravy of birds. Cooling diet is to be used in the two last forms; and in *Sitapita*, heating food is to be employed, and every thing cooling avoided.

TREATMENT OF ACIDITY OF STOMACH, VOMITING OF BILE, (*Amlapitta.*)

In this disease emetics are first to be used, followed by laxatives. When the patient has vomited, and has been purged, anoint his body with oil, and exhibit enemas. His food should be taken with bitter substances, but without any heating mixture. He should eat a preparation of barley and flour, and the powder of fried rice, with honey and milk. He should likewise take a decoction of the *Patal* leaves, ginger and coriander seeds, when there is much itching pain, and indigestion. When there is much fever and vomiting, accompanied with pain, take a decoction of the *Patal* leaves with ginger, myrobalan, and *Gulancha*. Tonics are also of great use, with carminatives.

TREATMENT OF ERYSIPELAS, CARBUNCLE ? (*Bisharpa.*)

When produced by air different preparations of ghee, and decoctions, and plasters are applied to the part. The medicines used are the same in all the above forms as follows:—take equal parts of

Musta,............(Cyperus rotundus,)
Sotáobha,.........(Anethum sowa,)

* Which consists of myrobalan, Emblic myrobalan, and Beleric myrobalan, mixed in equal proportions, or one tolá.

Debdáru..........(Pinus debdaru,)
Kusta,............(Costus speciosus,)
Kustumbru,.......(Coriander seeds,)
Cigruh............(Hyperanthera morunga,)

mix them with water and ghee, the mixture is then to be boiled, strained, and applied to the part. It is sometimes used as a decoction.

Stimulating medicines are likewise applied to the part, when the disease is produced by bile. The application in this form should be used cold. Thus take equal parts of

Bibera,
Lámojaka,
Chandana,
Rasanjana,.........(Sulphurate of Antimony,)
Gaerika,

mix them together with milk, and apply it to the part. In some cases cold water, or water mixed with honey or sugar, or the juice of the sugar-cane may be used with advantage.

When erysipelas is produced by phlegm the following medicines should be used. Take of

Ajagandá,...........(Ocymum gratissimum,)
Ashvaganda,........(Physalis flexuosa,)
Sahala,............. (Pinus longifolia,)
Tribrit,...............(Convolvulus turpethum,)
Ajasringi,

mix them with cow's urine to the thickness of cream, and apply it to the part. Another application is as follows. Take of

Kaláner sarga,
Agura ....(Aquilaria agallocha,)
Kachu,...............(Arum colocasia,)
Gunghá,..............(Morunga hyperanthera,)
Rásaná,
Bássau,..............(Panicum italicum,)
Sitasiba,
Indraparni,
Mahikadamba,
Pralendu,
Munjáta,............(Saccharum munja,)

these medicines are to be mixed with cow's urine to the consistence of cream, and then applied to the part.

Besides these external applications, purgatives, and blood-letting are recommended. When abscesses are formed, or the part ulcerates, the usual plan of treatment for abscesses, and ulcers is to be followed.

TREATMENT OF BOILS, PUSTULES, ERYSIPELAS? (*Bishphotaka.*)

The treatment of this disease is the same as that described under the head of (*Bisharpa*). The bark and leaves of the (*Sabanjana*) tree (*Morunga*) is to make into a paste with old conjee, and applied to the parts with salt; bitters are also of much use, such as the decoction of *nimba* bark and of *gulancha.*

TREATMENT OF SMALL-POX, (*Masùriká.*)

The treatment of small-pox is varied according to the humour particularly deranged.

The air pox (*Báyu Masùriká*) is to be treated by exhibiting the decoction of the powder *helamochee* with red sandal-wood. In other cases a decoction of

Gulancha,
Coriander seed,
Panchamùli,
Rásná,
Rátri.
Ushìrá, and
Durálabhá is recommended.

Two tolá of each medicine is boiled in a pint of water to ¼; this is given for a dose. The body is rubbed with ghee, mixed with a paste made of the bark of

Madder,..............Manjista,)
Bata,
Shirìsha,
Urumborroh, mixed together.

Kodeero (the leaves of Cakekim) and the leaves of *Nim*, are to be mixed, formed into a paste, and rubbed over the body.

When the small pox is situated in the mouth and throat, gargles made of

Subarnamákshyik, and
Dátrìfala, Emblic myrobalan,

are formed into a decoction and taken with honey.

When affecting the eye, the vapour of a decoction of wheat and liquorice is to be used.

When the pustules are broken and drying up, the powder of the ashes of cow-dung, and the ashes of astringent trees, as the bark of the *catechu* tree and *bata*, &c., are applied.

The diet in this variety of small-pox should consist of sweet articles of food with rice, and broth made of a decoction of peas.

The treatment of small-pox produced by bile (*Pìtta Masùriká*) is at the commencement, the decoction of

Nim bark,
Porpotoka,
Páta, *Patol*,
The red and white sandal-wood,
Ushìra, Hellebore,
Bássá, *Durálabhá*,

two tolá of each medicine, to two pints of water, which are to be boiled down to one pint. The decoction is to be taken in small quantities sweetened.

In small-pox produced by deranged blood (*Raktaja Masùriká*) blood letting, and the above decoction are required.

Small-pox produced by deranged phlegm (*Kapha Masùriká*) is to be treated by a decoction of bitter plants; and the body is to be rubbed with the bark of *shirìsha* and *urumborroh*.

The treatment of Measles consist in administering the juice of the leaves of *sushabì* with the powder of *haridrá*.

The preventative means to be employed in this disease are administering the powder of tamarind seeds with the powder of turmeric daily in cold water, by which means the person will not be attacked with the disease. The juice of plantain tree with white sandal-wood and water; or the juice of *Passo* with liquorice will have the same effect. These are to be given likewise when the fever comes to check, or diminish the violence of the disease.

In *Bhábaprakásha*, a modern compilation, another form of small-pox is related. It is called *shitalá*. In this compilation, antiphlogistic remedies are recommended to be used from the beginning; and the ashes of cow-dung is to be rubbed over the body. When the pustules have been broken, the person is to drink cold water, and he should remain in a cool room. Such a cool regimen, with an airy and clean place to reside in, is all that is required. Febrifuge decoctions are also used to diminish the fever, and various religious ceremonies, with prayers and offerings are used.

In other books the manner of treating small-pox varies according to its nature. In general, the treatment commences with rubbing ghee made hot, or warm water over the body, before the eruption appears; an emetic should also be given.

When the eruption makes its appearance the pustules are rubbed over with turmeric, mixed with ghee. Cooling food is recommended, particularly the powder of fried rice and gram, boiled with sugar and water. Broths made of the birds, which pick with their bills, such as pigeons, &c., are to be used towards the termination of the disease. Few people are allowed to visit the sick person; dirty people are particularly excluded, and no one is allowed to touch the person. It is said to be contagious.

TREATMENT OF DISEASES OF THE MOUTH, *(Mukharoga.)*

The diseases of the mouth are sixty-five: *viz*, eight diseases of the lips; fifteen of the gums; eight of the teeth; four of the tongue; nine of the palate, seventeen of the throat; and three general diseases.

Diseases of the lips.—When air produces diseases in the lips the treatment is to apply equal parts of goat's fat, sesamum oil, ghee, and wax, to the diseased part. Fomentations are also to be used to the lips. When ulceration takes place, apply frankincense, green rosin, (*dhuná*), a kind of gum (*gugulí*), and powdered liquorice. Mix and apply them to the ulcers in the form of powder. When the disease is produced by diseased bile, apply leeches and other local and general antiphlogistic remedies. When phlegm is diseased after local bleeding, use fomentations, gargles, and errhines, with fumigations. Powder of long and black-pepper, ginger, impure soda, nitre and black salt, mix them together with honey, and apply to the part.

When fat is diseased in the lips, foment, and if the lips ulcerate apply the actual cautery, after which apply powdered *pringí*, *ladra* and the three kinds of myrobalan: mix them together with honey. Such are the means of curing those diseases of the lips, which admit of being cured.

When the blood is deranged in the lips, the same treatment is to be followed, as when the bile is deranged.

Diseases of the Gums.—There are fifteen diseases described under this head.

Sitáda.—Remove blood by scarifications ; then use gargles made by decoctions of dry-ginger, mustard seed, and the three kinds of myrobalan. This mixture is to be used frequently.

Dantapapataka.—In the acute stage use scarifications ; after which mix rock, black, and common salts, *sachulla,* and *samberi,* with nitre and honey. Errhines should also be used, and food prepared with ghee.

Dantabeshta.—After scarifications use the following gargles : mix equal parts of the decoction of

Lodhra,............(Symplocos racemosa,)
Patanga,............(a kind of Sandal,)
Jastimadhu,.......(liquorice,) and
Lákshyá,............(lac,) or take honey, ghee, and sugar,

mix and apply to the part.

Sawesara.—After scarification apply a mixture made of the bark of

Lodhra,..........(Symplocos rocemosa,)
Mustá,...........(Cyperus rotundus,) and
Rasanjana ....(Sulphurate of antimony) with honey.

Other astringent barks may also be used in the form of decoction.

Mahásansira.—This form is to be treated as the last.

Parídarah.—This form is to be treated as *sitáda.*

Apakusa.—In the treatment use purgatives, emetics, and errhines. Scarify the part by rubbing the rough border of the fig, or other such leaves. Then mix the powder of long and black-pepper, ginger, salt, and honey together, and apply it to the part. As a wash use the powder of long-pepper, mustard, dry-ginger with tepid water. Prepared ghee with sweet and astringent medicines are to be used as a detergent.

Baidurba.—Any sloughing parts are to be removed with the knife, and the use of the caustic prepared from potassa. After which the antiphlogistic form of treatment is to be used.

Adìdanta.—When the air is deranged it produces irregularity in the growth of the teeth, with much pain; such teeth should be extracted, apply the actual cautery, and then treat it as of a caries of the tooth.

Adìmánsìka.—Scarify the swelled part, then apply powdered.

Bacha ....(Acorus calamus.)
Tejobatì,..................(Pothos officinalis,)
Páthá,..................(a sort of plant,) and
Sarjeká,..................(impure soda and nitre.)

Mix them with honey, and apply to the part. A powder of long-pepper mixed with honey may be used, and the wash of astringent and bitter decoctions is to be used frequently.

Susruta also states that there are five different fistulas connected with the gums.

In the treatment scarify the fistulous openings, and then use astringent and bitter gargles. Actual and potential cauteries are also to be used. Should such fistulæ be neglected they will extend to the bone, and the teeth should be extracted, and the part treated as a fractured bone.

If on removing the last molar tooth there occurs much hemorrhage, pain, and paralysis of part of the face, they prove that the tooth should not be extracted. When this has been done, use a decoction of

Játì,..................(Grandiflorum,)
Madana,..................(Mimosa catechu,)
Swádukantaka, and
Khadira,.................. Catechu.)

Diseases of the teeth.—Tooth-ache (*Dálana*), *Krìmìdantaka* or *worm eaten tooth.* The treatment should consist of stimulant applications, and oleaginous mixtures. If the tooth is loose it should be extracted. After the above medicine the actual cautery is to be applied to the diseased part.

Sensible teeth, (Dantaharsa.) For the cure of this disease apply hot ghee, and a decoction of medicines which cure diseased air. The application of the usual fumigations will be useful. The food should be animal broths, milk, ghee, and different preparations of rice, with oil to the head.

Dantasarkará.—In this disease remove the tartar, and apply powdered stick-lac (*laka*), with honey.

Kapáliká is cured by following the same treatment as the other varieties.

The following articles of food are to be avoided in diseases of the teeth ; acid fruits, cold water, hot, dry, and hard food, cleaning the teeth with a hard piece of wood, and not the soft recent branch of a tree as usually employed.

Diseases of the tongue.—When *air* is deranged in the tongue, the treatment should be the same as in the case of the lip produced by diseased air. When *bile*. the part is to be rubbed hard to discharge blood, and when the bad blood has been removed, sweet applications are to be used with collyria and washes for the mouth. When *phlegm* is deranged, the treatment should consist in rubbing the tongue with the rough leaves of certain trees, or by scarifications, and then applying to the part, the powder of long and black-pepper with honey. Water, in which the powder of mustard seed and salt have been mixed, is to be used for cleaning the mouth.

Apasìbá.—In this disease the tongue is to be rubbed with rough leaves to discharge the bad blood, and followed by the application of caustics, long-pepper, &c., mixed with honey. The powder of yellow mustard seed and white salt are to be boiled in water, and used as a wash for the mouth. Errhines and fumigations, will also be of great use in this disease.

Diseases of the palate.—Kantasunda (enlarged tonsils.) When they have become troublesome they are to be seized between the blades of a forceps and drawn forward ; and by means of a semi-circular knife the third of the swelled part is to be removed. If all be removed so much blood may be discharged as to destroy the individual. If too little is removed it will produce an increase in the swelling, with fainting ; a red secretion from its surface will be produced with sleepiness, an indistinctness of sight, swimming of the head, &c. After the operation, the part is to be rubbed with powdered black-pepper,

Alibissá,
Páthá,..............(a sort of plant,)
Bacha,................(Acorus calamus,)
Kushta,.............(Costus speciosus,)
Labana,............(Salt,)

mixed with honey. The infusion of several astringent herbs may likewise be used as a gargle.

Kachhapa, Raktabuda, Mánsasangáhta, Puputah, Tálupáka and *Tálushosh.* These six last diseases are to be treated by the use of the same medicines as the first. Fumigations are used for two days in the disease produced by deranged phlegm. The operations to be performed in the different forms of the swelling vary according to their nature. Sometimes a part of the diseased part is excised ; others require to be opened, others scarified, &c. The diet in all these forms of disease should be milk, and a decoction of *mudga* or pulse. In all these forms of disease cigars are made of those aromatic substances which are best suited to the nature of the disease, and smoked by the patient.

TREATMENT OF DISEASES OF THE THROAT.

Rahìnì.—In this disease the treatment is to bleed the patient generally and locally; give an emetic, apply fumigations, and use gargles and errhines.

When the *air* is deranged, after the discharge of blood, apply rock salt over the wounds, and warm ghee; fat, and marrow warmed are to be used as a gargle and retained in the mouth. This is to be repeated frequently.

Bile.—In this form, after bleeding, sugar, red sandal-wood, and honey are to be applied to the part, with a decoction of grapes and *Parusaka.*

Phlegm.—After bleeding, soot, mixed with hot articles, as long and black-pepper &c., is to be applied to the part. Oil prepared with

Siyatá,.........(Arabian jasmine,)
Biranga. and
Dantì..........(Croton polyandrum.)

to be used as a gargle.

When air, bile and phlegm are deranged at the same time, the treatment is the same as for the separate form. When blood is deranged, the treatment is the same as the last form.

Kantasáluka.—In this form scarifications are to be made on the swelling. The treatment should be the same as that of disease of the palate. *Ekabrinda.* In this form scarifications are to be made, and astringent gargles are to be used. *Gìlin.* It is cured by being removed by a knife.

In general the forms of disease, produced by bile should be treated by the antiphlogistic treatment, and those by phlegm by astringent and hot applications. When produced by air, the applications should be of ghee, oil, and other medicines for the cure of air.

TREATMENT OF DISEASES OF THE EARS, *(Karnaroga).*

In these diseases ghee is to be used with the diet, with rest, and bathing, not including the head, while intercourse with women is avoided. In *karnashùla*, *pranáda*, *bádhirjya*, and *kara* the treatment is the same. Give oleaginous purgatives, and apply steam of water impregnated with different herbs which cure air diseases. This is conveyed to the external ear by means of a tube. Fish, cock's flesh, and that of a bird called *lába* are to be mixed, and applied hot to the ear. The leaves of the banian tree, are to be made in the form of a cup, which is to be heated over a fire, and the drops of juice which ooze through the leaf, are to be applied hot to the ear. The juice of garlic and ginger is also to be applied to the external ear. Other stimulating and narcotic medicines, and different oils, are recommended for these diseases of the ear. Srong errhines are also to be used.

In deafness the oil is to be prepared with cow's urine mixed with a decoction of *billah*, and applied to the ear. Milk and water are also of use. For curing the diseases named *karnashrába*, *pútikarna* and *krìmikarnaka* are the same remedies as above enumerated. Strong errhines and fumigations, washing, oils dropped into the ear, aud various astringent decoctions will be found of use. Gum, raisin, frankincense *(dhuná)*, powdered with the juice of the wild cotton tree, are to be applied to the ear. Worms are to be removed by the application of such medicines as expel them. The sulphurate of arsenic, with cow's urine, is found of use. For removing the bad smell from the ear, use fragrant fumigations. Mustard oil will remove the ringing of the ears. Inflammations of the air are to be treated as in other local inflammations. For the morbid secretion of wax remove it by instruments, and fomentations; and emetics and errhines are to be administered for the itching of the ear. For removing external substances from the ear exhaust the air in a cow's horn, and apply it tightly upon the part.

In defects of the external ear, *Susruta* recommends the surgeon to prepare a new ear, by removing skin from the neighbouring part, leaving a connection to keep up its vitality.

Cutting off ears was a frequent method of punishment and the formation of a new ear removed the deformity.

TREATMENT OF DISEASES OF THE NOSE.

Pinasa, Putinaska.—In these diseases the treatment should consist in anointing, and heating the body. Then an emetic and purgative are to be given, and errhines exhibited. Hot food is to be used in small quantities, and of a kind easily digested. Boiling water is to be taken as soon as possible, and the part exposed to steam impregnated with aromatic substances. The powder of pepper, dry-ginger, &c., may be mixed with mustard oil and the urine of cows, to be boiled together, and used as an errhine.

In *Putinaska* ghee is to be introduced into the nostrils with fomentations. Emetics and errhines are also to be used, with light food, and warm water as drink. Smoking with aromatic herbs is also recommended. In this disease mustard oil is to be used; it should be prepared with the following medicines:—

Hingu,..............(asafœtida,) black and long-pepper, and dry-ginger,
Bachaka,
Shibati,
Katphala,
Lákshyá..............(Butea frondosa,)
Bacha.................(Acorus calamus,)
Kusta.................(Costus speciosus,) and
Biranga.

These are mixed, and used as an errhine.

Násíkápáka.—In this case antiphlogistic means are to be used, as the application of leeches, and the paste made of the bark of the trees which produce a milky juice, as the banian tree.

In *Puerakta*, when pus and blood are discharged, it is to be treated as fistulæ in other parts of the body.

In *Pinasa* hot substances are to be eaten, as ginger with salt, so as to thicken the mucus, and when chronic ghee is to be taken internally with emetics. When the mucus becomes thick it is to be discharged by means of errhines, purgatives, gargles, and smoking with aromatic substances. The person should remain in a shut up place. His head should be kept warm, and he should avoid cold water and venery. He should also avoid grief, dry food and new wine; when accompanied with fever, vomiting, languor, and diarrhœa, fasting is recommended with tonics and carminatives.

TREATMENT OF DISEASES OF THE EYES, (Akhirogah.)

Eleven of these diseases are cured by the excision of the diseased part; nine by scarifications; five by incisions; fifteen by punctures; twelve by the use of different instruments; seven are cured with difficulty; and fifteen diseases are incurable. The two general diseases of the eyes are considered incurable.

In treating Ophthalmia (*Abisanda*), the patient is to have his body anointed, and fomented according to custom; and in both *Adimanta* and *Adisanda* venesection is to be employed, followed by oleaginous glysters and purgatives. Cooling washes, and the vapour of certain medicines, with errhines, are to be applied to the diseased eye. It is then to be covered with a yellow-coloured cloth. Warm fomentations, and boiled hot flesh is to be applied to the eye, with poultices made of milk and rice. The patient should drink milk boiled with the decoction of those plants which cure diseased air. Goat's milk, boiled with the decoction of the root and leaves of the castor oil shrub is to be applied to the eye while warm.

When the ophthalmia is produced by derangement of the bile, blood-letting, purgatives, and the applications recommended in other inflammations are to be used. In other cases ghee and goat's milk are to be prepared with the following medicines. Take of

Gundrá...........(Cyperus pertenuis,)
Sháli,
Shaibala.........(Vallisneria octandra,)
Loclobido,
Dárbi...............(Zanthorrizon,)
Elá..................(Cardamoms,)
Udpoloh,
Rodhra,
Mustaka...........(Cyperus rotundus,)

and the leaves of the water-lily and other cooling medicines. Ghee is to be used as an external application. The other parts of the antibilious treatment is to be followed; and gold rubbed in the milk of a woman, and mixed with honey, may also be applied. Liquorice root, mixed with woman's milk or sugar and water; or a piece of cloth made of the wild silk is to be first moistened with water, and then applied to the eye.

When ophthalmia is produced by phlegm, blood-letting, fomentations errhines, and colleria, with the application of vapour are to be used. Different gargles, and irritants for the discharge of mucus from the nose are recommended. The colleria, &c., are to be prepared with medicines which cure phlegm. The patient should eat of such substances as do not increase phlegm, the ghee should be prepared with bitter plants. This should be repeated daily. The fomentations should be prepared with the decoctions of

Bálá............(Hibiscus tortuosus,)
Suntí............(Dry-ginger,)
Debdáru.........(Erythroxylon sideroxcylloides,)
Kushta............(Costus speciosus.)

The vapour of these medicines is to be applied to the eye. At other times various medicines are formed into a mixture, and applied externally to the eye: such as myrobalan, *haridrá*, (turmeric), *maduka*, (liquorice), *anjana*, and antimony. These medicines are dried in the sun, and when the mixture is to be used, moisten it and apply it upon the eyelids.

When blood produces diseases of the eye, it is recommended to use general and local bleeding, strong and frequent purgatives, errhines, cold applications, and to apply a mixture of different medicines upon the eyelids. When there is much pain use soothing fomentations, leeches, and the usual treatment for bile. The juice of *nimba* leaves mixed with iron and copper are also recommended. The juice of sugar-cane, honey, sugar, woman's milk, *darbia* and *maduka*, (liquorice), are to be applied externally, with the juice of the pomegranate. Water and sugar, rock-salt, and whey are also used as external applications.

Kukunáka.—In the *treatment* bleeding is first recommended with scarifications of the eyelids. Then apply stimulating substances mixed with honey, in order to discharge the bad humours. With this the usual medicines recommended for the mother and child, for purifying the humours and improving health are to be given; such as emetics, &c., are to be used. A decoction of the young leaves of *jumbu* (rose apple), *ámra* (mangoe), *datree mulica*, and myrobalan trees, are also recommended. The eyes are to be washed with this, as well as with other astringent medicines. The following mixture is also recommended. Take of

Nipálaja, (red sulph. of Arsenic), *maricha*, (black-pepper). burnt kunch, (a shell), *rasánjana*, (sulph. of Antimony), and *saindhaba*, (rock-salt), with jagry and honey. These medicines are mixed with the honey and treacle, and applied with a probe to the eye.

There are many peculiarities in the diseases of the eyes, that cannot be described in a book; but by these general precepts an intelligent person will be able to vary his treatment according to the circumstance of each particular case.

The diseases of the eye in which the use of instruments is required are :—

Utsinjini,
Bahalabàrta,
Hurdamabárta,
Shábabárta,
Bandabasta,
Klistabárta,
Pataka,
Kambíkini, and
Bátasarkárá.

Scarifications.—Before performing this operation the person should take an emetic and purgative. He should be placed in a closed cool room without much light, the eyelids separated by the thumb and forefinger of the left hand. Moisten the eye with a piece of soft cloth which has been dipped in warm water; and with the point of a knife on the rough leaf, as of the wild fig tree, &c., the scarifications are to be made. Continue the application of the warm water as a fomentation; after which the following mixture is recommended.

Take of

Manageh............(Red sulphurate of Arsenic,)
Káses...............(Sulphurate of Iron,)
Baso..................(Long and black-pepper and dry-ginger,) and
Saindhaba..........(Rock-salt).

Mix with honey, and apply a small portion with the probe to the inside of the eyelid. This is to evacuate more completely the bad humours. After these have been discharged the medicine is to be removed by bathing the eye with warm water. Ghee is to be applied to the eye. These applications are to be used, with the exception of the scarifications, every third day.

The effect of these scarifications on the inside of the eyelids is to stop the morbid discharge, to diminish the swelling and itching as the eyelid becomes smooth. Such results prove that the eyelid has been properly scarified. If not performed well, the following are the symptoms; the redness, swelling, and discharge, continue, and the symptoms of the disease are not removed. The eyelid becomes black, heavy, and is moved with difficulty. There is much itching and irritation in the eyelid; and sometimes it produces suppuration of the eye.

The nine diseases in which scarifications are to be used, are

Bortábabandá,
Clestabártang,
Bálabártang,
Patakí,
Sáhuburta,
Cardamaburta,
Cambikíni,
Sùkárá, and
Utsanjanì.

Incision of the eye should be employed in.

Bishagrantì.—In this disease fomentations are first to be used; when matter forms, open the abscess, and then apply powdered rock-salt with the sulphate of zinc, (*kásís*), long-pepper, red sulphurate of arsenic with honey, to the part, and put on a bandage.

In *Lágana* divide the parts and then apply the powder of *Ráchanás* (supposed to be the concrete bile of the cow), saltpetre, sulphate of copper, and honey. In other cases the actual cautery must be applied. Treatment of *Unjánámeká,* (styr), consists in fomenting the abscess, and then applying the sulphurate of antimony with honey.

For the cure of *Bishagranta,* first foment, open the part, and then apply the powder of the three kinds of *matabah, tuto,* (sulphate of copper), *kásis,* (sulphate of iron), and rock-salt. These medicines irritate, and increase the secretion of tears, and clear the organ. Then use astringent applications.

In *Upanáha* cut off the diseased part, and then apply fomentations; and a mixture of long-pepper, rock-salt, and honey.

Excision.—In *Udemánsarniá,* (Pterygium), excision is to be used for the cure of this disease. First mix ghee with the patient's food; then apply stimulating powder to the part, followed by fomentations. The eye is then to be rubbed with the finger, and when the eyelids are somewhat loosened apply a hook, and draw the fleshy growth; slightly outwards. Then pass a needle under the diseased growth ; tie it, and then separate the diseased part from the cornea and sclerotica with a round formed knife. Then apply fomentations and a bandage.

The only diseases in which excision is employed, are :—

Sírájála,
Sorbanícá,
Ursa,
Sarskársa Urbada.........(Small tumours.)

Pakakapat. (Intropeon). In this distressing disease it is recommended that from the inner to the outer canthus of the eye a portion of the skin is to be removed, about three times in breadth, in the lower third of the upper eyelid. This operation is particularly described by *susruta*, who states the kind of room which should be used as an operating room, that in which the patient is to be placed, his diet, &c. After the operation apply honey and ghee to the wound, which should be brought together by hair sutors. These are removed on union taking place. If this operation is not successful, destroy the roots of the hair by the actual or potential cauteries.

Amaurosis, (*timira* or darkness). The patient is first to get oleaginous purgatives prepared with old ghee which has been kept for some time in an iron vessel. The ghee is also recommended to be prepared from amphibious animals. It is to be rubbed up with water and applied to the eye ; different preparations of antimony are likewise recommended, such as antimony, honey, sugar, red sulphurate of arsenic, mixed together, and applied to the eye. Different colleria, fomentations, errhines and other external applications are also to be used. These preparations of antimony with other stimulants are to be used. Bleeding is not recommended, but errhines are highly extolled. Various other remedies with nutritive diet is recommended, as barley with much ghee, the juice of myrobalan, and the flesh of wild animals and birds.

Cataract, (*linganása*). In treatment of this and other diseases the patient should first take ghee, as it is supposed to cure the diseases of *air*, which are supposed to derange the other humours. The weather should neither be very hot nor very cold in which the operation is to be performed. The eyelids are to be kept properly separated by an expert assistant; the patient is then to be directed to look to his nose, and a knife with a point shaped like a grain of barley is to be held between the fore and middle fingers, and thumb of the right hand if the left eye is to be operated on, and in the left hand, if the right eye. The knife is then to be carried forward near the junction of the sclerotica with the cornea, neither high nor low in the eye, (near the transverse axis) and pass it on until water escapes. Then introduce a probe with a hook at its extremity, which is to detach and remove the cataract. When the person sees well, immediately after the operation, it has been properly done, particularly when the pupil appears clear like the other eye. After the operation apply the milk of a woman to the eye, with fomentations. Then cover the eye with a bandage. For ten days after the operation he must remain perfectly quiet in a dark room. During this time his food should be light.

In the treatment of the following diseases of the eye, the knife is not to be used:—

Sukákípáka,
Kaphabidagdhadristì,
Pittabidagdhadristí,
Sakra,
Urjana,
Pishtaka,
A'mlakí,
Akilnabarta,
Damadarsí,
Suktí,
Prikelnabarta,
Balásabasta.

In external injuries, and their consequences, the following diseases are cured by bleeding:—

Sírájála,
Siráharsa,
Nainapáka,
Pabanunátah,
Pucálása.

Also in acute and purulent Ophthalmia.

TREATMENT OF DISEASES OF THE HEAD, (*Síraroga*).

When *air* is diseased in the head, take ghee, milk, and

mudga (a kind of pea), and boil them in water: *máskalai* at night will also be useful. Avoid bitters, hot milk, warm baths and *douches* applied to the head. A hot poultice composed of fish, and the expressed oil of sesamum will be of use. It is also diminished by hot applications and bandages.

The smoke produced by oleaginous substances is to be applied, and the person is to anoint his body with prepared oil, and have errhines and purgatives exhibited. The juice of oleaginous substances mixed with the food, and with medicines useful for curing deranged *air*. Throwing warm water upon the head is often used, and sometimes the water is mixed with other medicines.

Bile. The pain is diminished when the head is kept cool, and during the night. Medicines are to be given with cold water, milk, ghee, oil, and the like, and applications are to be made to the head; as vinegar, the juice of the sugar-cane, of acid fruits, or whey. The paste of aqueous plants, purgatives, enemas made with oil, and broths made of wild animals are also to be used.

Phlegm. In this form the medicines which cure diseased phlegm are to be used, such as strong emetics, errhines, and gargles. The head should be rubbed with a paste made of liquorice root and ghee. The bark of *inquido* is also useful; and snuff made of the bark of *katfala*. He should likewise take the decoction of those medicines which cure phlegm, and live on rice and barley, mixed with long and black-pepper and ginger. The decoction of *mudga* (a kind of pea) may also be used.

When the above three *dhátu* are diseased, the treatment is the same as that above described, as being applicable when one only of the humours are diseased; particularly the use of old ghee internally.

When the disease is produced by a diminution of brain, or fat, phlegm or blood, in the head, nourishing food is to be used, with prepared ghee applied internally and externally. The prepared ghee recommended in pulmonary consumption is also to be used.

Worms sometimes produce severe pain in the head. The treatment consists in using medicines to discharge the worms; as blood, when used as an errhine, it will cause the worms to become stupid. Stimulating snuffs are of use, such as the powder of the seeds of *shringí*, and *biranga* mixed with cow's urine, and other vermifuge medicines. By these means the worms will be expelled.

Súrjyábartta.—For curing it use old ghee, and other medicines, as above mentioned; and the food is to consist of milk and rice, with broths made of wild animals.

Anantabáta.—This variety is to be treated in the same manner as *Sùrjyábartta* but particularly by the puncture of the diseased vessel. The diet should be sweet-meats prepared with ghee, honey, sugar, and flour, with the remedies which cure bile and air.

Ardháyabhedaka, (*hemiplegia*). In this form errhines prepared with the powder of the seeds of

Sirisa,
Mulaká.........Camphor,
Pipala..........Long-pepper, and
Bacha are to be exhibited. An external application is made by mixing together the paste of

Sáliba,
Kusta,
Pipala and *Madhuka*, (liquorice) with the juice of acid fruits, ghee, and oil. This is applied over the head. The broths of wild animals, with ghee, and cold applications, are also useful. The head should, in this disease, be always kept well anointed with mustard oil. If by the above means the head-ache is not checked, blood-letting should be performed.

Sank haka.—The treatment is the same as of the last variety.

TREATMENT OF DISEASES OF THE FEMALE ORGANS OF GENERATION.

The *treatment* of these diseases will vary according to the humour diseased.

When the *air* is diseased apply warm fomentations such as steam baths, &c., and poultices, use also injections of oleaginous and other medicines heated, which cure diseased air. A piece of cloth soaked in oil is to be kept in the vagina.

When *bile* is deranged with much bearing down and inflammation, use cold lotions. If there is a bad smell, use the decoctions of astringent barks.

When *phlegm* is deranged take the juice of garlic every morning, with food made of rice and milk, and apply different tinctures to the part, as recommended under the head of midwifery.

In dismenorrhagæa the patient should live on nourishing food, fish, *máskalái*, sesamum seeds (*til*), curdled milk, and drink cow's urine, whey, and wine. The pubis should be well rubbed with oil and ghee, and the vagina is to be kept distended by the introduction of a roller of cloth.

The treatment of menorrhagia should resemble that of hemorrhagia, such as the application of cold and astringent medicines, avoiding venery, and living on cooling and simple food.

Kanda, (*Utero Vaginal Tumours.*) For the treatment of these tumours use the flesh of shell-fish, and the pulp of tamarinds, rub them together, and apply the mixture to the tumour. A paste made with the flowers of *Gossa*, are to be applied to the part, and will be found of great use.

TREATMENT OF DISEASES OF INFANTS, (*Bálaroga.*)

An infant should have an aperient mixture once a month, in order to keep the bowels clear; and prevent his being affected with diarrhœa. Indeed, almost all diseases are produced by constipation.

A child sick within the month of his birth, is to have honey, milk, sugar and ghee mixed, and put on a piece of rolled cloth like a candle, which he is to be allowed to suck. The dose must be increased according to the temper, growth, and constitution of the child, until he is a year old. From 1 to 16 years the above will answer; and other medicines, of a stronger description should be employed according to the constitution, and nature of the sickness.

Errhines should not be given to a child under seven years, smoking under twelve years, medicinal waters to clean the mouth until the child has passed his fifth year, nor a brush to clean his teeth before his twelfth year.

When a pregnant woman continues to give suck to a child, it produces cough, bad appetite, vomiting, drowsiness, and emaciation. In this case the milk is to be changed, and tonics are to be given.

Tálukantaka.—In this case the mother's milk is not wanted, and very thin food is to be given in very small quantities, when the child is thirsty.

POISONS AND THEIR ANTIDOTES, (*Panata*).

Antidotes for Vegetable and Mineral Poisons.—In the first stage of the effects of these poisons, give cold water to drink, with an emetic. In the second stage, give an emetic with a preparation called *agada*. This medicine is prepared with ghee, and the following vegetable decoctions :—

Madaka............(Bassia latifolia,)
Tajara..............(Amaranthus,)
Kusta...............(Costus speciosus,)
Badradára........(Phrynium dichotomum,)
Haranu.............(Tróphis aspera,)
Pannúja,
Allá,
Albáluk,
Nágapuspa........(Bauhinia anguina,)
Utpala..............(Nymphœa cærulea,)
Sítíá................(Lycopodium phlegmaria,)
Balanga...........(Ocymum,)
Chandana.........(Sirium myrtifolium.)

Mix this with honey and ghee. Soon after a purgative is to be given. In the third stage give *Agada* internally as an errhine, and collyrium.

In the fourth stage give *Agada*, and ghee.

In the fifth stage give *Agada* with honey, and a decoction of liquorice.

The sixth stage is to be treated as a case of Dysentery.

In the seventh, errhines of *Agada* alone, are to be used.

In all the stages the antiphlogistic treatment is to be followed, with ghee and honey. *Conjee* water is also to be given, mixed with a decoction of

Kakátukì.........(Diospyros tomentosa,)
Agníka.............(Premna integrifolia,)
Pátá................(Sida lanceolaria,)
Surgíbalí.........(Cleome pentaphylla,)
Amertá............(Menispermum cordifolium,)
Abaycá,
Surísa............(Sinapis dichotoma,)

Kíníhí............(Achyranthes aspera,)
Sála...............(Shorea robusta,
Haridrá..........(Curcuma longa,)
Dár Haridrá....(Curcuma zanthorrhizon,)
Punanabbá......(Trianthema monogynia,)
Huranu,
Tríkatí............(Monetia barleroides,
Sáriba............(Periploca Indica,) and
Ballá...............(Pavonia odorata.)

Treatment of Snake bites.—When the extremities are bitten immediately apply a tight bandage above the bitten part. This may be a piece of cloth, a piece of leather, the flexible bark of a tree, or the like; so as to prevent the poison entering into the system. When a bandage cannot be so applied the bitten part is to be cut out. In all cases cutting out the part, sucking the wound with a horn, or burning the part is highly proper. When the mouth is used for sucking place a piece of bladder over it first, and then suck. Different prayers (*mantras*) are to be used as the bandage is applied; but a scientific man should not rely on *mantras*, as other means should be used, as antidotes, &c., to prevent the effects of the poison. When the poison has reached the head, the person should be bled; and cold water prepared with *Chandana* (Sirium myrtifolium, a fragrant wood), and *Usíra* (Andropogon muricatum, a cooling root), is to be used for bathing, and internally the different antidotes are to be given mixed with honey. If these antidotes are not at hand, give the black earth of ants nests, or *Sirisa* (Mimosa Siris), and *Karbudára* (black-hellebore); and avoid spirits or wines. Fluids that cause vomiting are of use, as the poison is thus removed from the system. If these means do not succeed, then bleed the person, and give *Azida* with honey and ghee. The errhines and collyria are likewise of use, when made of different antidotes. In the fourth stage give emetics, followed by barley corn for food. In the fifth and sixth stages use an antiphlogistic treatment, and in the seventh give strong errhines, as ammonia, &c.

The above treatment is applicable to the other, as well as to the hooded-snake bites; but when the class of *Rájíla* serpents have inflicted the bite, bleed, and then give the antidotes as above mentioned. When the treatment is not successful, and the person is insensible, make a crucial incision on the crown of the head, and apply to it a piece of recent flesh of an animal; then exhibit errhines, make a loud noise to rouse the person, and when his senses return give him a strong purgative. The antidotes should be continued for some time after the symptoms have disappeared, otherwise the violent symptoms will be liable to recur.

The following are varieties of *Azída*, or mixtures of antidotes for the cures of poisons, particularly of snakes. Take of

Trivrit.........(Convolvulus turpethum,)
Bishalá.........(Aconitum ferox,)
Madaka.........(Bassia latifolia,)
Haridrá......(Curcuma longa,)
Dára Haridrá(Zanthorrhizon,)
Raktá..........(Nymphœa odorata,)
Arjúna........(Terminalia alata.)

The five salts, with long-pepper, black-pepper, and ginger powder, are to be mixed with honey, and kept in a close vessel. They are to be given internally in water, and used at the same time as a collyrium, and errhine. This is considered as the most efficacious antidote known.

The following is an antidote for animal and vegetable poison:—Take of

Bíranga.........(Verbesina prostrata,)
Pátá................(Sida lanceolaria,)
Trifolá..............(The varieties of myrobalan,)
Ajamodá,
Hingu............(Asafœtida,)
Chakrá.............(Citrus decumanus,)

Mix with black-pepper, long-pepper, dry-ginger, and the different kinds of salt. Reduce them to a powder, mix them well with honey, and keep them in the horn of a cow. This is to be shut with a piece of *pith*, and keep it so for a month. It may be used as an antidote for animal, vegetable, and mineral poisons. It is called *Azìta*, or never failing antidote.

Different other varieties of these antidotes are given in *Sushruta*, &c., but these two are considered the most efficacious.

Poisonous rats.—When they discharge their semen upon any part of the body, the blood is affected, and produces different glandular, swellings, blotches, and eruptions. In these cases *Sirisa*, (Mimosa Siris), and *Kusta*, (Strychnos Nux Vomica), are to be taken internally, with impure potassa made of the wood *Palása*. In these cases bleeding is recommended with purgatives and emetics. The parts first touched by the poison are to be burned or scarified, and over the part a mixture of *Sirisa*

(Mimosa Siris), *Rajani* (Cleome corocana), *Kusta*, (Strychnos Nux Vomica), *Kunkuma* (Crocus sativus), and *Amrita* (Menispe rmum cordifolium), is to be applied.

The Bites of Mad Dogs, Jackals, &c.—In all cases the first part of the treatment should be to scarify the part, and squeeze out the blood, after which the part is to be burnt by means of hot ghee. Then apply to the wounded part *Azída*, or a mixture of antidotes, and give old internally. Errhines are also to be given with the milk of the *Arka* plant, (Calotropis gigantea). Apply also the *Sitá*, *Punarnabá*, (Trianthema monogynia), *Dhatura*, (Datura metel), or the flesh of animals; and *Til* oil, jagry, milk of *Rupiká* mixed and applied to the wound. By such means the poison may be destroyed soon after the infliction of the wounds. In other cases take two *tolás* of the following root—

Sharapunkhá...........(Trophis aspera,)
Dhatura...............(Datura metel.)

Let one *tolá* be mixed with flour of rice and water, and wrap up in the leaves of stramonium. Roast it into cakes, and give it to the patient. The quantity is not stated. After taking this medicine other bad symptoms may occur, which may however disappear without any other remedies. During the treatment the patient should be kept in a cool situation, without any water. When the symptoms disappear the person should then bathe, and on the third and fifth days the above cakes are to be administered in half the dose given at first. He is then to take rice and milk. It is recommended in these cases to act powerfully on the system by strong medicines, before the poison has produced its constitutional effects. After the infliction of the wound, and before it has produced any constitutional effects, the free use of water in bathing is recommended, and the bowels are to be afterwards opened by purgatives and emetics, followed by errhines to clear the passages.

Scorpions.—In mild cases apply oil (*Chakartaila*); warm water prepared with *Bidari*, (Gmelina Asiatica), and other sedative vegetables. Apply to the part a poultice made of the antidotes, the powder of turmeric, salt, long and black-pepper, dry-ginger, and *Sirisa*, (Mimosa Siris). It is also recommended to apply the juice of the lemon, cow's urine, with the leaves of *Sirisa*; or apply cowdung after it has been heated. Give internally honey with ghee, or milk with sugar, or cold water with sugar, and different kinds of *sharbats.*

Spiders.—The part should be cut out, and the actual cautery should be applied to the wound. The part is then to be rubbed with honey, and salt, or *Azída.* The person is also to have purgatives, and emetics administered to him; and should there be much swelling, apply leeches. In all the varieties of spider-bites apply *Azída* to the part.

Emetics for Poison.—Drink goat's milk, after the poison has been taken, until the person vomits; this is to be repeated until it does not produce this effect, when no more poison is present. Black coloured poison is never to be used as medicine.

Hemp, (*Gánjá* or *Grinjá*).—For preventing these effects, ghee, the juice of the sugar-cane, raisins, sugar, water and honey are recommended; after sour articles have been given to produce vomiting. The mouth is to be washed with sweet, sour, and bitter substances, which will improve the senses, and its effects on the heart; and the bad particles of the poison which get into the brain will be discharged. For doing this more effectually, as is supposed, incisions are sometimes made into the crown of the head, with the fanciful intention of discharging the pernicious smoke. During the cure hot articles of food are avoided, and light food and ghee, and the like is proper.

Dhatura............(Datura metel,)
Amrita..............(Aconitum,)
Ahìphena............(Opium,)
Karabíra root........(Nirium odorum,)
Arka..................(Calotropis gigantea,)
Lánguli..............(Gloriosa superba.)

All these poisons are purified by being boiled in hot milk, or in water mixed with cow-dung for half an hour; and the kernel of the seed is generally used internally, mixed with other stimulating medicines. Thus *Joypal* (Croton seeds), when it has been so boiled, is mixed with pepper, vermilion, and other medicines. This mixture is given in small doses in the beginning of fever. Datura is prepared in this same way, mixed with other medicines and used as a narcotic and stimulant. Euphorbium (*Sìhunda*), and the root of the Abrus precatorius, Oleander (*Karabìra*), Hellebore (*Kataki*), and the different varieties of aconitum are prepared by reducing the roots to small pieces, soaking them in cow's urine, and three days before it is to be used removing it from the liquid; dry it in a strong heat, and administer it at first in doses the size of a mustard seed, increasing it for seven days, and then diminish the dose. A leprous person may take one *gunja*, which is about the weight of one *rati*, or one and a half grains. When this poison has been administered in too large doses give goat's milk, which will produce vomiting, and thus remove the poison from the stomach. The dried bile of fish, of goats, buffaloes, wild boars, and peacocks are used, and are administered as stimulating medicines. These five varieties of bile are much employed as stimulants. They are purified by being macerated in the juice of lemon. (These different poisons with croton seeds are the chief ingredients in the celebrated "*bis bari*" or poisonous pills.)

Nux Vomica (Kusta, Kupilu) is prepared by being steeped for three days in *conjee-water*. It is then mixed with mustard oil and other medicines, and is used by the moderns as a powerful internal medicine in small doses, and as an external application for the cure of leprosy.

Bitumen (Silájatu), Petrolium (Boomutylum), are got in hills in which gold and silver are found. It has the smell of cow's urine, and is bitter, salt, and cold. It is usually mixed with different other medicines, is supposed to have an alterative effect, and may be advantageously used in the cure of all diseases.

The most common manner in which it is employed is as an external application in rheumatic complaints, and in cases of epilepsy, hysteria, and palsy.

Poisons should be taken internally in the quantity of a mustard seed for the first day, and increase it for seven days, adding the same quantity each day. For the next seven days a quantity equal to a mustard seed, is to be given less each day. The third week a quantity equal to a barley-corn in size is to be administered, and increase one each day for seven days; and the fourth week each day one less is to be given for seven days. No more is to be given unless in cases of leprosy when the size of a *rati* is to be given. Poison is to be taken with milk, it is not to be given to very hot-tempered persons, to those with deranged bile, to eunuchs, or to patients with bloody-sputa. When the person has a great appetite, or is very thirsty; when greatly fatigued, when any of the humours (*dhátu*) are weakened during pregnancy; in the house of a *Rájá*, or when there is a violent quarrel with the patient and another person, poisons must not be used in the treatment of diseases.

The mineral poisons may likewise be used in a diluted form as medicines. Such as the

Rasa-carpura.........(Corrosive sublimate,)
Gadanta................(Yellow orpiment,)
Tuta.....................(Sulphate of copper.)

The last poison is prepared as a medicine in the following manner. Mix it with half its weight of sulphur, expose it to heat for two hours. It may then be used in medicine, and it will neither produce vomiting nor giddiness. The other poisons when prepared so as to diminish their power, may be employed with advantage in the cure of many diseases.

The *weak poisons*, such as

Akunda.........(Asclepias gigantea,)
Segdutra.........(Euphorbia,)
Bislánguli......(Nama zeylanica,)
Karabìra.......(Cleome pentaphylla,)
Gusinga.........(Rondeletia cinerea,)
Dephena.........(Saliva of serpents,)
Noki.........(Pontedera vaginalis,)

and other sweet smelling drugs. These are divided according to their colour and form, as like animals, ears, &c. They are mixed with cow's litter, honey, and conjee; are boiled, or made into a powder. They are to be washed in pure water, and dried in the sun.

None of the above poisons should be given to a person under ten, or above eighty years of age. The teachers should take a dose, so as to remove the fears and doubts of the pupils.

TREATMENT OF DHAJABHANGA OR CLAIBA, *(Impotence.)*

For this disease different kinds of nourishing food and drink are to be used; the patient is to live in a good house, indulge in good beds, in music, in the society of beautiful women, in wines, and in perfumes, as all these tend to remove sterility. The medicines to be used are as follows: Take of the powder of *Bìdárì* or of *Anuloka* mixed with honey and ghee; and eat the testicles of goats roasted and prepared with salt, ghee, and long-pepper. The preparations of *mashkalái* and sugar, barley, wheat are also of use. The eggs of crabs and of crocodiles, or of turtles properly prepared will be of great use. Flour prepared with ghee, and milk, and rubbed on the feet with oil, prepared with crocodile's eggs; the flesh of rats, frogs, and the eggs of sparrows are recommended. The patient is to drink fresh milk with sugar, honey, and powder of *Swayanguptá* and *Ekuruka*.

TREATMENT OF GUDABHRANGSA, (Prolapsus Ani.)

The treatment to be pursued is to foment the part, apply oleaginous substances to the prolapsed gut, and return it slowly. Then a bandage is to be applied, on which a convex piece of hard leather is to be placed over the anus, and retained there by means of a bandage tied round the loins and between the legs. Fomentations are to be occasionally exhibited, and the body of a rat from which the intestines have been removed, is to be made warm and applied to the part effected. Milk and a decoction of *Mahá Pankamúla* are to be given. The decoction is to be strained, and exhibited internally and externally.

TREATMENT OF AHIPUTANA, (Superficial Ulcer round the Anus.)

These ulcers are to be treated by exhibiting purgatives, and other medicines, to purify the milk of the mother. Then give a decoction of tonic medicines to the child consisting of *Patala-patra*, the three kinds of myrobalan, with prepared ghee. These are to be given internally. Locally, astringent decoctions are to be applied, and the sulphate of zinc (*Kapalatuta*) is to be sprinkled over the ulcers.

TREATMENT OF EMACIATION, (Kársa.)

The person should use milk, ghee, animal and sweet articles of food, with barley, and flour. He should sleep in the day time, avoid venery, and not work much. The powder o, *poischia*, *asuganda*, *bidárì*, *shatábarì*, *balla*, and *nágaballa*f are used as tonics, with alteratives.

TREATMENT OF UNHEALTHY (Costiveness) Discharges, (Amaha.)

The treatment is the same as in *Udábarta*.

TREATMENT OF WOMEN DURING PREGNANCY AND LABOUR.

From the time of conception the woman should be happy, she should remain pure, should wear ornaments and white clothes, and the names of the *gods*, *guru*, and *bráhmans* should be frequently repeated and worshipped. Such a female must not touch dirty, diseased, or imperfectly formed individuals. Things with a bad smell, and every thing bad, or disagreeable to the sight, are to be avoided; she should avoid fasting, the use of dry articles of food, food prepared the day before, or putrid, or food that had been moistened. This last remark refers particularly to rice. The female should remain at home in order to avoid devils, and avoid houses in which the possessors have died; or enter temples, or where bodies are burnt, or under trees. Anger also is to be avoided. She should avoid fatigue, venery, carrying heavy weights, sleeping in the day time, watching at night, grief, blood letting, or violent exercise, as horse exercise. She should live on well boiled, and easily digested food; is not to speak loud, or exert herself so as to be fatigued, which may affect the fœtus; should not besmear the body with oil, or turmeric. Her bed should be soft and low. Such food is to be given as she wants, but it must be soft, thin, sweet, oleaginous, and what promotes the internal heat. Such directions are to be observed until she is delivered. During the three first months the food should be very sweet, cool, and thin, as rice and milk; the fourth month she should take curdled milk; the fifth milk; sixth ghee; and during the seventh month ghee with milk, prepared with a decoction of *Prutuck purnee*, &c., should be given, as it will retain the fœtus happy, and nourish it. During the eighth month give enemas with a decoction of

Badara,..............(A kind of plum,)
Balá,..................(Pavonia odorata,)
Atibalá,................(Annona squamosa,)

with milk, whey, oil, and ghee. By this means the bowels are cleared, the air will be retained in a favourable state for assisting at the delivery of the infant, and will ensure its proper position. After these enemas give barley or rice, with the juice of wild animals.

The woman is to be removed on the 9th month to the room in which she is to be delivered. This is generally a temporary shed built for the purpose near the house, and is afterwards destroyed. The removal must be on a favourable day. The house in which a *Bráhman* woman is to be delivered must have a white floor; a *Khetriya* woman a red floor; *Baishya*, yellow floor; and a *Sudra*, a floor of black earth.* The house is to be made of *Bel* wood, if the woman is a *Bráhman*; if a *Khetriya*, the wood of the sacred (*Nyagrodha*) fig tree; the *Baishya* house

* The emblems of the degree of purity of the individual.

is to be made of the *Tendraka* tree, and for the *Sudra* of the *Bablá* tree. The house and cot are to be made of the same wood, the walls must be clean, and the furniture properly arranged. The door should be either to the east or south, and eight cubits long by four broad.

The approach of delivery is known by the descent of the uterus, and the more flaccid state of the abdomen, the breasts become relaxed, and pain commences in the loins, back, and inside of the thighs. When it is approaching, pain is felt in the sides and back, there is a frequent inclination to stool, and mictirition, followed by a mucous discharge from the vagina. She should have male children to surround her bed, and she should hold in her hand flowers and fruits of a masculine kind. Her body is to be well anointed with oil, and bathed in warm water, and then sour gruel is given in large quantities to assist by its weight and quality in expelling the child. The bed is to be soft, with high pillows under her head, she is to lie on her back, her thighs are to be separated, and her legs bent. Four old experienced women are to attend. They should have short nails, and know the art of delivering; and before whom the patient has no shame or fear. When labour has commenced, these women must tell the patient that her infant, like an extraneous substance, must be expelled, and that the proper time has arrived. The patient must be directed to press downwards, by retaining her breathing so as to expel the fœtus during the pains, particularly when the pain extends to the buttocks, inside of the thighs, abdomen, and pelvis. When the head of the child is near the osexternum the mother must try with all her force to expel the child.

The patient must be careful not to force downwards at an improper time, as in such a case the infant will be deaf and dumb, its cheek bones will be crushed, and the head deformed. The child will also cough, breathe with difficulty, its body will be dried up, hump-backed, and ugly. These are the consequence of the undue pressure. Should the child advance crooked it is to be turned straight by manual assistance.

If the infant be retained in the passages an unusual time, apply smoke to the vagina of the skin of black serpents, or (*Pindítaka*) a kind of tree. She should also tie some of the root of the

Hirunnopusbei.........(Similax glabra,)

Bitullá....................(Cicer arietinum,) or
Subjachillá...............(Sabia lanceolata,)

round her arms and leg, to promote the expulsion of the fœtus.

When the infant is born, a little fine salt and ghee are to be mixed, and a small quantity put into its mouth. A mixture of bruised *nim* leaves (Melia azadirachta), aud ghee are to be rubbed over the head, and a piece of oiled cloth put over it. The umbiliacal cord is to be tied with a string, eight fingers breadth from the navel, and then divided; and one end of the string is to be bound on the neck of the infant, to prevent evil. A little cold water is next to be thrown upon the face of the infant, and the father offers up the prescribed prayers, and a mixture of honey, ghee, *Anantá* (Bromelia Ananas), and the juice of the *Bramhí* plant (Ruta graveolens), is to be mixed with the powder of gold, and a piece of it is to be placed in the infant's mouth; or these medicines are to be given with a golden spoon (Menu, p. 21, ch. 2, s, 29.) The body of the infant is to be anointed with oil, and washed with the infusion of the bark of such trees as have a milky juice. In other cases fragrant infusions are used for washing the infant, or water heated by the immersion of hot silver or gold, according to the circumstances of the father and state of the fœtus.

Should the secondines not be removed, the abdomen remains tense, swelled, and painful, and the dejections constipated. In such a state a finger covered with hair is to be introduced into the throat of the mother, so as to produce vomiting, when the secondines will be expelled. In other cases disgusting substances are given for producing the same effect. In other cases the smoke of different articles are applied to the vagina, such as wild pumpkin, mustard seed, the skin of serpents, with sour milk, oil, &c. Other articles are applied to the vagina for the same purpose, as the root of the *Kusta-langulí* (Nama zeylanica), and alvine evacuations mixed with urine, and wine. These are boiled in white mustard or ghee, oil is to be added, and the mixture is rubbed over the belly.

The first milk of the mother appears about the fourth day, and is to be thrown away; and as much as can be retained in the palm of the hand is to be mixed with honey and ghee, and given to the infant at two periods. After this the child should obtain nourishment from the mother.

After delivery the mother's body should be anointed with oil prepared with a decoction of *Ballá* (Terminalia bellerica), or a decoction of such articles as remove an excess of air. Should any excess of air, bile, or phlegm exist, long-pepper and its root, *Hastì-pippulí* (Arum macrohizon), *Chitraka* (Limonia pentagyna), *Seringabera* (Quercus lanceofolia), are to be powdered, mixed with water of treacle, and given warm. For two or three days this is the only food to be given, or until the bad blood is removed; and when it is purified, give a decoction of rice and barley gruel, prepared with *Bedáríganda* (Bauhinia variegata ?) and other plants, with milk. This decoction is to be continued for three days; then give rice with the juice of wild animals. This regimen is to be continued for 15 days, or until the mother's strength is restored. After this period, she will leave the temporary house in which she was delivered, and return to her usual occupations.

If the woman does not observe these rules of diet and regimen after delivery; but lives on improper or poor food, exercises herself too early after delivery, exposes herself to fatigue or to changes in the weather, she is liable to other and dangerous diseases; such as fever, diarrhœa, dysentery, anasarca; and in other cases to pain, costiveness, weakness, dyspepsia and all diseases produced by deranged air and phlegm. These diseases after parturition are called *Sutiká-roga,* and are cured with much difficulty, or when the woman is weak they are incurable. These are likewise produced by grief, and when they have occurred, they are to be treated according to the custom, nature, place, and age of the patient; and when judiciously treated, she may be cured.

After delivery the body is dry, if hot things are given, and bad blood remains, and is collected by the air in the uterus, it produces swelling in the umbiliacus, sides, and in, and above the bladder; with great pain in the pelvis, head, and breast, as if these parts were pierced with needles. In other cases it stops the urine, and is accompanied with fever, pain over the body, thirst, shivering, heaviness, and causes swelling of the abdomen and dysentery. This disease resembles *Makalah.*

Certain decoctions, such as *Biratarù* (Sida cordifolia) are given for the cure of this disease, as also the powder of nitre, with warm water, and ghee. Powdered long-pepper, and other such articles, with wine, are also given.

These are the complicated and dangerous diseases.

TREATMENT OF THE INFANT.

The infant is to be covered with silk cloth, and the bed should be properly made, and of soft materials. It is to be fanned with the branch of a *Nimpilu* tree, is to have the oiled cloth daily applied to its head and face, and always kept in the room with the mother. The room is to be smoked with a mixture of several sweet-scented gums and woods, accompanied with a suitable prayer. White mustard seed is to be thrown round the child to prevent the approach of evil spirits, and such charms are to be applied to the neck, head, arms, and legs as will prevent their approach. Linseed and mustard seed are also to be sprinkled over and around the infant for the same purpose. After ten days the father and mother, with the prescribed ceremonies, are to name the child according to their pleasure, or the star which is in the ascendance at the time of birth. During this time the parents are to remain pure and happy.

Wet Nurse. The nurse should have a perfect body, of a yellowish tinge, be neither long nor short, neither lean nor fat, of a middle age, without disease ; of a good temper, of a stayed good disposition, and without covetousness. The milk should be good and flow easily from the nipple, which should not be long, not too large, nor too small, nor the mammæ large. If good the milk will be cold, clean, white, like a white shell, should mix with water without bubbles of air, and should not be glutinous.

When the woman is very hungry, is grieved, fatigued, has bad humours, is again pregnant, is feverish, very thin, or very stout, and eats roasted things and unhealthy mixtures ; or when the nipples are not long, and the mammæ large and pendulous, the milk will not be so good.

The nurse should have pleasure in children, if not, the milk will dry up soon. She should not work at a low occupation, and should be of a good family. The more of these qualities the nurse possesses the better. A fortunate day is to be found out upon which the infant is first to get the breast. Before this is done the nurse is to bathe, and have new clothes given to her. She is then to sit down with her face towards the east, with the child's to the north. Then the right mammæ is to be washed, and a little milk removed. If the breast is given the child without this precaution the milk produces difficulty of breathing, coughing, and vomiting.

This is to be avoided, and the next milk given with a prayer, for an abundance of good milk, which will afford strength, and health to the infant, like that of the gods. If these directions are not observed, and the milk of different nurses given, diseases will be produced in the child. The nurse must avoid heavy things, must eat her food at regular intervals, and avoid whatever will derange air, bile, or phlegm ; as this will render the milk bad, and produce diseases in the infant. She also should avoid bad mixtures and situations, such as anger, grief and care, as by these means the milk is diminished and rendered unhealthy. To increase the milk she should be encouraged, and made happy. For this purpose she should live on nourishing and easily digested food, such as barley, flour, rice, the broths of animals, fish and good vegetables.

If a nurse uses bad food, her milk is affected, and produces pain and derangement in the humours of the infant. A good physician should observe the signs of all such diseases. The infant, if pained in a part, will touch it frequently, and if it is pressed it will cry. If the head be diseased, the infant will keep his eyes closed, and he will not be able to support the head. If the bladder be diseased the urine will be suppressed with pain, thirst, and faintness. If the urine and dejections are discoloured, the colour of the body is unnatural, with vomiting and swelling of the abdomen. When the air is accompanied with noise in the intestines and crying, the whole body is affected. In such cases give soft and mild medicines, with the milk of the mother or nurse. The medicine which will soon cure deranged air, bile, and phlegm is to be used. If milk is given alone to the infant, any medicine that may be required to be given during this time must likewise be given to the nurse.

If the infant lives on milk and rice, the nurse is to take medicine at the same time ; but should the child live on rice alone, medicine is not to be given to the nurse when the child is diseased. If upwards of one month old, and the child live on milk, a pinch of medicine is only to be given ; if it live on milk and rice, the dose of medicine is to be of the size of a stone of a plumb. If only rice, the size of a plumb is to be given.

If the child lives on milk, the medicine is to be formed into a paste, and applied to the mother's nipple. If such a child is affected with fever from diseased air, milk is alone to be used for several days. To give ghee on the first day is improper. When fever accompanied with thirst is present, the mother's milk is not to be given. Vomiting and purging are improper in such cases, unless when the symptoms are very severe. If the abdomen is swelled at the navel, with pain, medicines to cure air will be proper; such as anointing the part with oil or ghee, and proper fomentations. If near the anus, and suppuration occurs from diseased bile, the antiphlogistic treatment is to be used. Such as the external and internal use of the sulphurate of antimony.

The child is to be moved about gently, the expression of loud noises is to be avoided, and he is not suddenly to be awoke, nor be moved quickly, as it will derange the humours. He is not always to be kept sitting, lest his back becomes humped, on which account he is to be moved about, and pleased by every means. Avoid exposing the child to wind, to the sun, or to lightening. He is not to be placed under trees, especially when creepers are upon them, in empty or bad houses, and in low places. Shadows of houses are very bad, and the glare of lamps is to be avoided; as also bad things of the same kind. The parents must avoid the influence of planets, of demons, by the usual ceremonies and customs. Unclean places, elevated or unequal situations, or when there is much heat, wind, dust, smoke, and water are to be avoided.

If the mother or nurse's milk is not good, use goat's milk; or if not to be got, cow's milk; but do not give much at a time. At six months give light and good rice, with the usual ceremonies, and the child must be kept clean. When epidemic diseases rage in a place, remove to another, but be careful to avoid places haunted by bad spirits.

If any kind of devils enter the child, it will be sorrowful and fearful, and always crying, and is sometimes senseless. The nails and teeth are used in snatching, biting, and grinding his teeth. He is always gaping, and the eye-brows more upwards and downwards, and the eye is directed upwards. He foams from the mouth, and bites his lips. What is eaten passes undigested, he breathes with difficulty, has no sleep at night, and is weak. The surface of the body remains flabby, and the smell of the body is like that of the feet, of the musk-rat, or bugs. Sometimes he takes the milk of the nurse, and at other times it is not wanted.

When the child's strength and intelligence have increased, about the fifth year, his studies must be commenced, and will be regulated according to his caste and condition. The marriage state should not be consummated before the twelfth year in the female, and twenty-fifth year of the male. If a male before the twenty-fifth year has a child with a woman before the sixteenth year, the offspring will die in the uterus; or if it is born alive, it will not live long, or if it lives, the mental as well as bodily organs will be defective. Connection is to be avoided with very old or young males or females, or those who labour under chronic diseases.

MEANS OF PREVENTING ABORTION.

Abortion is threatened when there is severe pain in the uterus, loins, groin and bladder, and blood is discharged from the vagina. In such cases the effusion of cold water and cold bathing is to be used, and cooling things are to be applied to the surface of the body. Internally milk and ghee, prepared with the class of medicine called *Geboneo* are useful; or that which preserves life. If the movement of the infant be considerable, exhibit milk prepared with *Utpoládí*. If the pain is severe, with a discharge of blood, costiveness and retention of urine, or the displacement of the fœtus, give oleaginous medicines internally, and apply them externally. If the pain is very severe take milk prepared with the decoction of

Mahasia.........(Jessaminum pubescens,)
Kudrosia........(Paspalum scrobiculatum,)
Moduko...........(Phaseolus mungo,)
Sodonstrá........(Tribulus terrestris,) and
Kantikárí.......(Solanum jacquini.)

Mix with sugar and honey. If there be retention of urine, give milk prepared with diuretic decoctions, if the costiveness is severe give asafœtida, *Sauburechullá* (a kind of salt); *bach* (orris root), prepared with milk. If there is much discharge of blood give the following mixtures:

Kostágáruká..........(Corchorus capsularis,)
Somongá................(Triticum æstivum,)
Dátukí..................(Andropogon,)
Nabamálika.........(Webera tetrandra,)
Guerìka..................(Leucocephala graminifolia,)
Sargarasa............(Brassica rapu ?)
Rasánjana............(Sulphurate of antimony,)

mix these with honey. In other cases a mixture of astringent medicines is given, the antiphlogistic diet and treatment followed, and a piece of cloth soaked in astringent decoctions is to be stuffed into the vagina. If abortion is thus prevented, the female is afterwards to live on a strict diet, consisting of milk prepared with a decoction of *Urambara* (fig). Boiled rice and barley, without salt or ghee, is also to be given. If there be much pain in the belly give old jagry with other carminatives. Sometimes by deranged air the fœtus is retained more than ten months, which will destroy it. In such cases the mother should have nourishing food and oleaginous medicines, such as broths made of the flesh of *Utkrosa* (a bird), with ghee and rice, &c. In like manner the mother should exercise herself, particularly in raising and lowering her head and body, as in humming, &c., and should ride over a place which has inequalities on its surface. If the air dries up the fœtus, the belly does not enlarge, and the fœtus moves little about. Iu such cases strengthening broths, and other food with milk is to be used. Sometimes the fruit of the conception is removed by the influence of devils. In such cases the symptoms of pregnancy suddenly disappear.

Food during the different months of Utero Gestation.

The food of the mother should be regulated so as to prevent abortion. During the 1st month give

Jastimadhu......(Liquorice,)
the seed of the teak tree,
Sáka poisa.......(Centaurea muschata?) or
Kirkákoli,.........(Cucumis utilissimus,) and
Sùrádáru..........(Phyllanthus ramnoides,)

in a decoction with milk.

2nd month. *Asantaka*......(Terminalia alata,)
Tila.............(Momordica monodelpha,)
Pipulí.........(Ficus religiosa,)
Tammarabuli(Tamarindus Indicum,) and
Sataguri......(Nelumbium speciosum,)

in a decoction prepared with milk.

3rd month. *Berkáduni*.........(Asclepias rosea,)
Kirkákoli..........(Cucumis utilissimus,)
Anantá............(Justicia adhatoda,)

as before, with milk.

4th month. *Anantá*........(Justicia adhatoda,)
Sumálá........(Sarcostema viminialis,)

Ráshná.........(Dolichos sinensis,)
Padá..............(Nelumbium speciosum,)
Maduka.........(Bassia latifolia,)

as above.

5th month. *Beruti*.........(Volkamerea infortunata,)
Kantikárí.....(Solanum jacquini,)
Kássari.........(Enonymus tingens,)
Kirisung.......(Butea frondosa,)

(the roots and bark of banyan, or *bot* tree) prepared with ghee and milk.

6th month. Decoction of
Pristapurní ?
Ballá..............(Pavonia odorata,)
Sigru..............(Hyperanthera moringa,) with milk.

7th month. *Siringátakah*...(Quercus lanceofolia,)
Minála............(Erythrina suberosa,)
Drákshya.........(Grapes,)
Kaseru............(Enonymus tingens,)
Maduka...........(Liquorice,)

and sugar mix, and prepare the decoction with milk.

Should abortion threaten, more milk is to be added to the medicines.

8th month. *Kapittah*..........(Dolichos pruriens,)
Birátì................(Volkameria infortunata,)
Balla.................(Pavonia odorata,)
Patala...............(Trichosanthes laciniosa,)
Ikkhu,...............(Saccharum officinale,) and
Kantikárì,.........(Solanum jacquini.)

The roots of these medicines are to be boiled, and used with milk.

9th month. Liquorice,
Anantá,......(Justicia adhatoda,)
Kirkákoli,...(Cucumis utilissimus,)
Sádibá,........(Rosa glandulifera,)

are to be given in the form of a decoction with milk.

10th month. Milk with dry-ginger and *Kirkákoli* are to be boiled together. If pain is felt in the stomach take dry-ginger, *Jastimadhu* (liquorice), which are to be boiled together. By these medicines pain will be prevented, and removed, and the child will be nourished.

If the woman becomes pregnant six years after the first pregnancy, the second infant will live a short time. If severe and dangerous disease occur during pregnancy, mild medicines mixed in sweet and sour vehicles are to be given; with soft, digestable, and nourishing food, as rice, milk, &c. If emetics or purgatives are required, give them of the mildest description. At the same time medicines are to be given, when the air, bile, and phlegm are deranged. The medicines as well as the food should be given weak, particularly the former.

The following four mixtures are to be given to the infant to increase his bodily strength and understanding.

1st. Take gold well powdered,
Kusta root......ditto,
Bach root........ditto,
mix and give with honey and ghee.

2nd. Take.
Muchakúka,......(Pterospermum suberifolia,)
Sankapuspi,......(Vinca parviflora,)
and powdered gold. Let them be mixed with honey and ghee.

3rd. Take.
Arkapushpa,......(Calotropis gigantea,)
Bach,................(Iris germanica,)
and powdered gold. Let them be mixed with honey and ghee.

4th. Take of
Katfala,..........(Hedychium gracile,)
Sítá,...............(Anethum sowa,)
Durbá,............(Arundo bengalensis,)
and powdered gold, mix and take with ghee and honey.

Preternatural Parturition, (Múrhagarbha.)

Is divided into

1. *Kíla* or *Breech presentations.*

2. *Pratikhara*, when a hand, foot, or head present, and the body is fixed.

3. *Bíjaka* is when one hand presents with the head.

4. *Parigha*, when the infant's body lies transverse.

In some manuscripts it is stated that this is not a proper

division of the different presentations. There are many other kinds, sometimes the hands present, sometimes the knees, some times one knee, in other cases the knee and side of the body, sometimes the side and back of the body, sometimes the two hands and the head, and sometimes the fœtus is situated across the mouth of the uterus. In some cases the mouth, sometimes the anus presents, which are always dangerous. In other cases when the woman becomes senseless, is affected with nervous diseases, and there is a contraction, or any disease of the vagina or uterus, parturition is always difficult and dangerous.

The fœtus may die in the uterus, by great grief or other passions; by injuries of the abdomen, by eating very hot things, or by diseases of the child. Such causes will naturally separate, and thus destroy the child, as worms and storms destroy the fruits of trees.

When this takes place the signs are the cessasion of the movements of the child, the absence of the peculiar pains of labour, the livid colour of the face, the fœtid smell of the breath, and pain in the vagina. When abortion takes place within the four first months, when it has received a soul, it is called *Garbhabichyuti;* should it occur after this period, when the parts are all perfect, it is called *Garbhapâta.*

When air is deranged in the abdomen or vagina, severe pain is experienced, and it produces *Mutrakrichchhra,* (Strangury). Monsters are produced by the sinful actions of the parents, and twins are produced by the air in the uterus.

Under ordinary circumstances, parturition is promoted by the action of the air, but when the air is deranged it produces unnatural presentations, and unusual parts of the child present, and it is impeded in its birth. When a prominent blue vein appears upon the abdomen of the mother, or when the body is very cold, and the mother is without shame, the fœtus will die. Both mother and child will die, when she is attacked during utero-gestation with a bad disease.

When the child dies from any cause, or delivery cannot be accomplished by the ordinary means, the woman is always to be considered to be in a most dangerous state. The woman's protector, whether a husband or father, and the *rájá* of the place is to be told the state she is in, and that the only hope the practitioner can hold out to save the mother's life, or give a chance to the infant being preserved, is the performance of a difficult and dangerous operation: as it is performed on an internal organ, in which the position of the child is liable to change, and is in the dark.

There are three cases which may impede delivery.

1st. By a deformity of the head.
2nd. By the shoulders presenting.
3rd. By the thighs presenting.

Should the infant be alive in the abdomen, the mother should try to expel it herself. If she cannot do that, prayers are to be repeated over some water which the woman is to drink, calling on the gods to produce natural delivery. As this prayer is pronounced, and the water drank, the various medicines for facilitating the expulsion of the child are to be given, while she lies on her back, with her legs bent, and the loins somewhat elevated. The hand of the practitioner is to be well covered with ghee, and introduced into the vagina, and thus remove the infant. Should the thigh present, the feet are to be brought straight together by the hand introduced into the uterus, and the infant thus extracted.

If the breach presents it is to be pushed upwards with the hands, and the legs extracted first. If the fœtus is transverse the lower part is to be pressed up, and the upper is to be brought down, and thus delivered. Should the side of the body or shoulder present, they are to be pushed upward, and the head is first to be delivered. If both hands present, push them upwards, and bring the head towards the vagina. The two last operations are performed with much difficulty. If it cannot be thus removed, the knife is to be used. If the hand cannot be so employed, the body of the infant is to be divided, and thus removed in pieces; but this is never to be done when the infant is alive, as by this operation both will be killed.

When a pregnant woman, near the full time, is suddenly killed as a goat is killed before the alter, and should the child move in the uterus, an incision is to be made in the abdomen, and the infant removed.*

* A case occurred, in which delivery could not be accomplished, and the child was alive, the physician told the husband that unless an operation was performed bath would die. It was referred to the woman, who with heroism answered, do not mind me, have the life of my child ! The operation was performed, the wound in the abdomen sewed up, and both child and mother recovered.

If the dead child cannot be removed the knife is to be used. The woman is to be encouraged with hope by kind language, and the (*Mundalágrá* or *Unglí Shástra*) knife is to be introduced through the vagina, the head is first to be divided, and the bones are to be separated and removed. A hook is to be fixed in the orbit or cheeks, and it is to be extracted. Then the hook is to be fixed in the breast, belly, or axilla, and the child is to be thus removed. If the infant be dead, and the shoulders present first, divide them at the shoulder-joint, and then deliver. When the abdomen of the fœtus is much swelled divide it, remove the intestines, and extract. If the breech presents, divide the bones of the pelvis and extract. In this manner any part which impedes labour is to be divided, and removed, so as to save the mother. For this purpose much care is required. As soon as the fœtus is known to be dead, a skilful practitioner will lose no time in completing delivery, as the woman will die very soon if the dead fœtus is left in the uterus. A pointed instrument should not be employed in performing this operation, as it is liable to wound the mother.

If the secondines do not come away, they are to be removed, by manual assistance. The abdomen is to be gently pressed on each side, and the patient is to be shaken by a strong person seizing her behind, after oil has been applied to the passages.

When the fœtus and secondines have been removed the woman is to have tepid water thrown over the body, and it is then to be anointed with oil, and a piece of cloth dipped in oil is to be applied to the external parts, which will diminish the after-pains, and keep the parts shut. After this give the mother the following mixtures to diminish the after-pains, and to disperse the bad humours collected in the part. A mixture of long-pepper, ahd its root, dry-ginger, asafœtida, cardamum seeds,

Byághrí.........(Eicus Indica,)
Jawání.........(Hedysarum alhagi,)
Bach.............(Iris Germanica,)
Atibisha.........(Annona squamosa,)
Rassia............(Dolichos sinensis,) and
Chaba.............(Cicer arietinum,)

which is to be given in powder with ghee, as a decoction or as a paste, This is to be repeated daily for three, five, or seven days, according to circumstances. Mild tinctures and wines are to be given at night. If any other disease appears at this period, the usual treatment is to be followed. The parts are to be washed with a decoction of

Círìsa.........(Achyranthes aspera,) and
Kakuba.........(Diospyros melanoxylon.)

The body must be kept perfectly clean. She should live on light milk food, and use daily warm oleaginous frictions, with the hand. Numerous prepared oil are used after parturition, till four months after. The patient should avoid anger, use milk with medicines which diminish air, for ten days. She may then take broths. If the strength and appearance of the body is completely restored, she is to return in four months to her usual diet.

VARIETIES OF MILK.

When the woman eats flesh, or other heavy food, it deranges the air, bile, and phlegm; and acting on the milk, produces various kinds of diseases in the infant. When milk is deranged by air, it is sour, astringent, and does not mix with water. When bile deranges it, it is of a yellow colour, bitter or sour, of a saltish taste, and it is thick, sinks in water, and is like mucilage when the phlegm is deranged. When two or three are deranged their individual appearances are found.

Good milk.—Mixes in water, is of a grey colour, like white smoke, is sweet to the taste, and has no sediment. Such are the qualities of healthy and nourishing milk.

SCIENTIFIC CATALOGUE OF THE PLANTS.

It gives the Bengali name, the medical or economical properties, date of introduction and flowering season, and whether or no the fruits are ripened, also the description of the Plant, whether shrub, tree, &c.

আখরোট *Ukrot.* Tree. Extends from Greece and Asia Minor, over Lebanon and Persia, probably all along the Hindoo Koose to the Himalayas. Abundant in Cashmere, Sirmore, Kemaon, Nepal, Assam, and the Khassya Mountains. Introduced into Honorable Company's Garden in 1795, but had not flower up to 1814. *Walnuts* are imported into Bengal from Cashmere, the Himalayas, the Khassya Mountains, &c.

আখরোট *Ukrot.* Large tree. Moluccus, Malay Islands, South

Mahratta country about Belgaum, Bengal (Serampore) Assam. Flowers small, greenish-white, hot season. Fruit. Aug. Kernels eatable, tasting like fresh walnuts. They yield by expression a large proportion of very pure, palatable oil.

অগুর *Ugoor.* Agallochum. Aloe's wood, Agila wood, Eagle wood. Large tree. Mountainous tracts E. and S. E. of Sylhet. Flowers small, greeen, March and April. Fruit rainy season, contains a fragrant resinous substance of a dark colour. It is considered a cordial by some Asiatic nations, and has been prescribed in Europe in gout and rheumatism, (Ainslie).

অঙ্গুর গাছ *Angoor gachh.* Shrub and climber. Country round the Caspian Sea, Armenia, Caramania; cultivated in India. Flowers small, greenish, February and March. At Serampore good grapes are to be had in April and May.

আচ *Uch.* A small tree. Common in most parts of India (Serampore). Fowers small, white, and fruit nearly the whole year Bark of the roots used to dye red. The colour is fixed with Alum, but it is neither bright nor durable. The green fruits are picked by the poorer class, and eaten with their curries. The wood is hard, very durable, variegated with red and white, and employed for gun-stocks in preference to all their kinds, (Roxb).

অড়র *Urur.* A shrub. Ceylon, both Peninsulas of India, Bengal, (Serampore) Assam. Flower largish, and fruit cold season. Cultivated. The seeds (দাল *dal*) are much esteemed by us. Cattle greedily eat the tender parts of the plant, whether green or dry; the dry wood is excellent fuel, and well adapted for producing fire by friction.

অনন্তমূল *Ununto-mool.* Shrub and climber. Ceylon, Coromandal, Malabar Hill, Bombay, Mazagaum. Abundant on the Hills at Wurgaum, Bengal, (Serampore) &c. Flowers 2⅓ line, on the outside pale green, on the inside, dark blood coloured. Rainy season; fruit rare. The roots are used as an excellant substitute for Sarsaparrilla. It is employed particularly for the thrush in children, giving about a dram, every morning and evening of the powder fried in butter.

অন্তমূল *Unto-mool.* Shrub and climber. Peninsula of India, Bengal, (Serampore). Segaen, &c. Flowers 5½ lines in diameter, externally pale greenish with a faint tinge of purple, internally light-purple, May and June; fruit August, September and October. The roots are used on the coast of Coromaudel, as a substitute for ipecacuanha. It is employed, as an emetic, by rubbing upon a stone 3·4 inches of the fresh root, and mixing it with a little water for a dose. It generally purges at the same time. Dr. P. Russel was informed by Dr. J. Anderson, the Physician General at Madras, that he had many years before known it used both by the European and Native troops, with great success in the dyseptery which happened at that time to be epidemic in the Camp. (Roxb).

অন্নানাস *Anannas.* Perennial. W. Indies. Domesticated in the Mascarenhas Islands, the E. Indies, Guinea, &c. Flowers small, bluish, hot season; fruit rainy and cold season. Pine-apples succeed as far north as 30° in the open air, but are plentiful in the garden of the Tajmahal at Agra. They are so abundant in Ceylon, parts of Burma and the Khassya Mountains, as to appear wild there and are considered most delicious in the two latter places. It is evident, therefore how well suited the climate and soil of many parts of India are to the cultivation of the pine-apple. This is important not only on account of the fruit, but also on account of the fibre, which abounds in the leaves, as with it cloth has been manufactured as fine as some muslins. (Royle).

অপাঙ্গ *Upanga.* A biennial. Both peninsulas of India, Bengal, (Serampore,) Nepal. Flowers small greenish, and fruit nearly the whole year.

অমলকুচি *Umul-Koochi.* Large shrub and climber. Peninsula of India, Bhagulpore. Flowers largish, yellow. In Honorable Company's Garden. Flowers rainy season. Fruit cold season. From the seeds is expressed an oil, which in some parts of the country is used to burnt in lamps. (Roxb.)

অম্বল বেল *Umblo-bela.* Perennial. Peninsula of India, Bengal, (Serampore). Flower small, May.

অরস *Urus.* A shrub. All over India, N. Holland, America. Flowers five lines, white, green-veined, and fruit the whole year.

অলাট চান্দন *Ulatchandul.* A perennial. Ceylon, Coromandel, Guzerat, Concans, Mahableshwur, Tavoy, Bengal, (Serampore) Morung. Flowers large, from the base to the middle first yellow, then blood-coloured, from thence to the apex blood-coloured, rainy season; fruit cold season. The root is said to be a violent poison.

অশোক *Ushok.* Coromandel, Ram Ghat, Martaban, Khassya

Mountains, Assam. Flower smallish, orange-scarlet. during the night fragrant, March and April; fruit August and September.

অশ্বগন্ধা *Ashwa-Gunda.* A shrub. Coromandel, both Concans, Guzerat, Bengal, (Serampore). Flowers $3\frac{1}{2}$ lines, pale greenish, rainy and cold season; fruit hot season.

অশ্বথ *Ashwuth.* পিপ্পল *Pippul.* Large tree. common all over India. Fruit receptacles axillary, paired, sessile, depressed, the size of a small cherry, appearing hot season; ripening rainy season. Birds are very fond of the fruit, eat it greedily, and often drop the seeds in cracks of buildings, where they vegetate occasioning great damage if not removed in time. *Wood* light and of little use.

আকন্দ *Akundo.* Flower beneath whitish with a tinge of lilac, above whitish light purple, with the crown purplish lilac, inodorous, or nearly so.

আকাশ বল্লী *Akash Bullee.* Perennial and twining plant. Mollucas, Ceylon, both peninsulas of India, Arabia, Bengal (Serampore). Flower small, white cold season; fruit February.

আকুশ *Aukkush.* Shrub and climber. Coromandel, Bengal, (Serampore). Flower small, greenish yellow; hot and rainy season; fruit rainy season.

আগমকি *Agumuki.* Perennial and climber. Both peninsulas of India, Bengal (Serampore), interior of the mountains N. India. Flower small, yellowish; and fruit throughout the year.

আর্জুনি *Arjooni.* Large tree. Bengal, jungles in the S. E. of Surat. Flower small. greenish-white, April and May; fruit December. *Timber* good, *Bark* in great repute among Indians as a tonic interally, and a vulnerary applied externally. It is sold by most Druggists. (Dr. Gibson.)

আটকে কলায় *Atke-Kulay.* মুগ ফল্লী *Moong Phullee.* Annual. Hot parts of America, domesticated in Africa, Asia, and S. Europe. Flower small, bright-yellow, rainy and cold season. Fruit February. The pods, which grow under ground, are sold in the Bazars. Seeds eatable, tasting somewhat like almonds or nuts, and used as a common article of diet in S. America. A sweet oil which does not turned rancid, is expressed from them, and an agreeable orgeade prepared from their paste, mixed with water and sugar. (*A Richard.*)

আমলি *Amli.* তিন্তুড়ি *Tin-tooree.* Tamarind tree. Molluccas, Both Peninsulas of India, Bengal, (Serampore), Assam. Flower middle-sized, somewhat orange, streaked with scarlet, slightly sweet-scented, May and June. Fruit, January and February. Wood durable, hard, beautifully veined. Leaves eaten in curries. Pulp of the fruit slightly aperient. Kernels, like those of the mangoe, eaten in times of scarcity and famine; reduced to a fine powder and boiled they form a tenacious paste, and a strong wood-cement, if thin glue is added. (Roxb.) The paste, simply smeared on the skin, has the property of rapidly promoting suppuration in indolent (blind) boils. (Wight).

আমুরা *Amoora.* Large tree. Soonderbuns. Flower small, yellow. Has not flower here.

আম্ব হলদী *Ambo-Huldee.* A perennial. Hindustan. Flower small, dull dark-pink, the lower segment of the inner limb tinged with yellow, and the tuft deeply coloured, rainy season; fruit none.

আম্লা *Amla.* Large tree. Moluccas, Coromandel, Concans, Deccan, South Mahratta country. Bengal, extending northwards to the banks of the Jumna. Cultivated in gardens. Flower minute, greenish-yellow, hot and rainy season. Fruit cold season. Wood hard and durable, particularly under water. Bark very astringent, used for tanning. Fruit succulent, sharp, unpalatable, unless pickled or preserved with sugar.

আলকুশী *Alkushee.* *Cow Itch.* An annual and Twining plant. Moluccas, both Peninsulas of India, Bengal, (Serampore,) Assam, Kheree Jungle, Deyrah Dhoon. Flower large, dark purple, cold season. Fruit hot season.

আলগোসা *Algosa.* An annual. Bengal, (Serampore). Growing on the lower parts of the stem of crotalaria juncea. Flower small, white, February and March; fruit April and May.

আশফল *Ash-Phul.* A tree. China, Cochin-china, both Peninsulas of India, Khassya Mountains, &c. Flower small, yellow-white, February and March; fruit April and May. Aril of the fruit not very grateful, but reckoned wholesome. Wood hard, close-grained and white.

আশ শেওড়া *Ash shoura.* A shrub. Peninsula of India, Bengal, (Serampore). Flower small, white, fragrant; fruit rainy and cold season.

persons) every half-hour till general discomfort is produced, when the worms soon appeared. To infants it has been found preferable to give twice a day, half a tea spoonful of the expressed juice of the young roots, mixed with a table spoonful of curds (দই) and a little sugar, till the worm is expelled. The flowers and the rind of the fruit are tonic and astringent, and as well as decoction of the bark of the root, used in dysenteric and other affections of the bowels. (*Trans. Med. Phys. Soc. Calcutta, Vol. I. p.* 363-64 B, *flore pleno.*) Flowers double.

আম *Am.* Large tree. All over India, thriving northwards up to Nahn, alt. 4000 F., but its fruit does not ripen there. Flower small, greenish-yellowish, February and March; fruit May, June, and July. *Wood* dull grey, porous, pretty durable if kept dry, but soon decaying by exposure to wet. In very large old trees, it acquires a light chocolate colour towards the centre of the trunk and larger branches, and is there hard, closer grained and much more durable. From wounds in the bark issues a soft, reddish-brown gum-resin, hardening by age and then much resembling Bdellium. Fruit too well known to require more than to be mentioned. Kernels large, seemingly containing much nourishment, but only used during times of scarcity and famine, when they are boiled in the steam of water and eaten. (Roxb.)

আমড়া *Amra.* Large tree. Peninsula of India, Bengal, (Serampore). Valleys of Deyra Dhoon and Kyarda. Flower small, white, March; fruit December and January. Fruit, when ripe, eaten raw; unripe it is pickled, put in curries, made into tarts, &c. From wounds in the bark a large quantity of a pure gum exudes, which soon hardens into a substance like gum arabic.

আমেক্লৌকা *Amclouka,* A shrub. Peninsula of India, Bengal, (Serampore). Flower small, yellowish, March and April; fruit June, July and August.

আমরুল *Amrool.* A small tree. Malay Islands, cultivated. Flower largish, greenish-white, hot and rainy season; fruit rainy season.

আমাদা *Amada. Mangoe-Ginger.* Perennial, Guzerat, The concans, Bengal, (Serampore). Flower smallish, white or pale-yellow, with a deeper yellow line running down the middle of the lip. The tuft, pale purple or rose-coloured, latter part of rainy season; fruit none. Root used medicinally.

আতা *Ata.* Custard-apple. A small tree. No doubt a native of tropical America, notwithstanding St. Hilaire's resonings, which would make it of Asiatic origin. No Anona has, on any good authority, been found wild in Asia, and it is perhaps, questionable, whether A. seneglensis, grandiflora and amplexicaulis, are true natives of senegal and Madagascar. Completely domesticated in India. Flower largish, yellowish green, hot season; fruit July, October, delicious. *Leaves* with a heavy smell. *Seeds* acrid, fatal to insects, and therefore it is powdered, mixed with *gram* flour, and thus occasionally used for hair washing. The fruit has, on some occasions of famine literally proved the staff of life.

আঁতমোড়া *Antumora.* A small tree. Extends from one end of India to the other, particularly along the foot of the Himalayas, (Serompore). Flower largish, brick-coloured, rainy and cold season; fruit February and March. Fruit used in dysenteries and bowel-complaints. At Bombay it is employed medicinally in diseases of the ear.—(*Dr. Gibson.*)

আদা *Ada.* আদ্রক *udruk. Common Ginger.* A perennial. Universally cultivated over all the warmer parts of Asia, but where indigenous, is not known. Flower small, whitish-purple, rainy season, but very rare. Seeds seldom perfected on account of the great increase of the roots. Extensively cultivated in the Himalayas, at the elevations even of 4.5000 feet in moist situations; in Bengal, the Bombay Presidency, &c. The root is dug up in October and November in other situations in February and March; the outer rind being rubbed off by various processes, the root is dried in the sun, and then called শুঁট *Soontha.*

আদা বর্ণি *Ada-burni.* A perennial. Flower smallish, blue, rainy and cold season; fruit cold season. Expressed juice, mixed with petroleum is employed to rub on parts affected with rheumatic pains. (Roxb.)

আনার *Anar.* ডালিম *Dalim.* Common Pomegranate tree. N. Africa cultivated in India. Flower large, scarlet and fruit at different periods of the year. The roots of this tree were already known in the time of celsus as a remedy against worms, but, have since 1804 performed such wonders in this respect, that they may almost be considered specific against tape-worms; two ounces of the bark of the dried root, cut into pieces, are boiled in a pint and a half of water till half a pint remains, four table spoonsful of the strained decoction are then given (to grown-up

আশান *Ashan.* পিয়াশাল *Piysahal.* Large tree. Monghyr, Rajmehal, Oudh. Common on the ghats and in the Concans. Flower small, greenish-white, April, May, and June; fruit cold season. Timber very valuable. Much used for making shafts of Gigs and other things where toughness of fibre is required. (Dr. Gibson.) Bark astringent and dyeing black.

গুঁড়ি কচু *Goori-Kuchoo.* আশু কচু *Ashoo-Kuchoo.* These two varieties are cultivated in Lower Bengal, about Calcutta, Serampore, &c. Small offsets from the larger tubers are, like potatoes, planted about the beginning of the rains, in May and June, in a well laboured, friable, rich soil, not subject to inundations.

ইন্দুর কানি পানা *Indoor-Kanee-pana.* An annual. Bengal. In Honorable Company's Garden flower rainy season. (*Roxb.*)

ইসফগুল *Issufgool.* An annual. Persia. Cultivated in India. Flower small, whitish, and fruit cold season. Seeds of a very cooling nature, and, like those of Plantago Psyllium, L., forming with boiling water, a rich mucilage, which is much used in India in catarrh, blennorrhœa, and affections of the kidnies. They are also deservedly recommended in chronic diarrhœa, two teaspoonful of them being given twice a day with a little powdered sugar-candy. (Ainslie-Twining).

ঈশ্বরমূল *Ishwur-Mool.* Shrub and climber. Rangoon, Penang, Coromandel. Cross-Island, Bombay Harbour. Hills throughout the Concan, Bengal, (Serampore.) Hindoostan, New Holland. Flower largish green, brownish red, rainy season; fruit cold season. *Root* nauseously bitter, considered to possess virtues against lues menostasia.

উক্ *Ook. Sugar-Cane.* Produces sugar. Arab, *sukkur*; Hind Jagry. A perennial. E. and W. Indies, Society Islands. Flower rainy season. The juice of the sugar-cane is the best antidote to arsenic. (Chisholm.)

উচনতি *Oohchunti.* An annual. Belgaum, Bombay, Bengal, (Serampore.) &c. Flower small, pale purple, cold season; fruit March. Has an unpleasant smell.

উচ্ছা *Oochhya.* Annual and climber. Cultivated. Flower middle sized, pale yellow, rainy and cold season; fruit cold season.

উড়ুজাতি *Oodoo-Jati.* A shrub. Flower 2 inches, livid-verdigris, coloured, with a white tube. Common in most parts of India and flower nearly the whole year.

উলকি পানা *Oolki-pana.* An annual. Bengal. In Honorable Company's Garden flowers rainy season.

উলট কম্বল *Oolut Kumbul.* A small tree. Moluccas, Interior of the Peninsula of India. Flower middle-sized, dark-purplish brown, hot and rainy season; fruit cold season. *Bark fibres* tough, adapted for cordage.

উলু *Ooloo.* A perennial. Caucasus, New Holland, Moluccas, Ceylon, both Peninsulas of India, Bengal, (Serampore), &c. Flower rainy season; fruit cold season. In Bengal much used for thatch.

একতীর *Ekteer.* A perennial. Bengal, (Serampore), Mauritius, Bourbon, St. Domingo, Jamaica, Guiana. Flower rainy season.

একবীর *Ekbeer.* A perennial. Bengal, (Serampore), Peninsula of India, Moluccas. Flower rainy season.

এলাইচ *Elaich* এলাচী *Elachee.* A perennial. Hilly parts of Malabar, and Travancore. Introduced at Poway in Salsette. Cultivated about Soonda Soopa, South of Dharwar. Flower large pale greenish-white, with the lip marked chiefly in the centre with purple-violet stripes. Was introduced into Honorable Company's Garden in 1809, but had not flower up to 1814. Produces the well known *cardamums.*

ওড়চাকা *Orchaka.* A small tree. Soonderbuns, Martaban rivers, Penang, Singapore, Malacca Straits, Salsette, Delta of the Indus, &c. Flower large purple. In Honorable Company's Garden flower hot and rainy season; fruit cold season. (Roxb). It is probably identical with the "*Tewar,*" noticed by Dr. Heddle in his Mss.

Report on Scinde, as being a better substitute for coal in steamers, than any other kind of wood. The supply stated to be inexhaustible in the Delta of the Indus. (*J. Grah, l. c.*)

ওল *Ol.* Moluccas, Ceylon. Both Peninsulas of India, Bengal, (Calcutta, Serampore,) &c. Flower minute, June. This species, which deserves to be called the Telinga Potatoe, is much cultivated in the N. Circars and about Surat, and highly esteemed for the wholesomeness and nourishing quality of the roots. A very rich soil, repeatedly ploughed suits it best. The small tuberosities found in the large roots are employed for sets, and planted in the manner of potatoes. In twelve months they are reckoned fit to be taken up for use; the larger roots will then weigh from 2-4 or more seers and keep well if preserved dry.

In the Kainah Zillah, it is planted in May; and yields from 100-250 maunds per beegah. It sells for about a rupee per maund.

ওবা চাঁপা *Ova-Champa.* A large tree from the Khassya Mountains, introduced in Honorable Company's Garden before 1814, is not easy to say. It is mentioned neither in Wall. Cat., nor in Royal. Ill., and to Mr. Griffith, who is familiar with Bhutan, Assam, and the Khassya Mountains, it is entirely unknown.

ককজঙ্ঘা *Kokojongah.* A shrub. Lower Bengal. (Serampore.) Flower small, greenish, rainy season; fruit cold season.

কর্কী *Kurkkee.* A perennial. Bengal, Peninsula of India Flower rainy season.

কঙ্কানটি *Kunka-Nuti.* লালনটি *Lal-Nuti.* An annual. Bengal, (Serampore.) Flower minute, greenish and fruit rainy season. Cultivated as a pot-herb by Bengalies. Sometimes it is called it বাঁশ পাট লালনটি *Banspata-lal-nuti.*

কঙ্গিয়া *Kungiya.* Large shrub and climber. Khassya Mountains. Flower middle sized, purple, March and April; fruit cold season.

কঙ্গু *Kungoo.* An annual. Cultivated. Flower rainy season; fruit cold season. Seed an article of diet.

কঙ্গু জুড়িয়া *Kungoo-Jooria.* A perennial. Bengal, (Serampore.) Flower and fruit rainy season.

কঙ্গুয়া *Kungooya.* An undershrub. Ceylon. Peninsula of India, Bengal (Serampore.) Flower smallish, rose coloured, rainy season; fruit cold season.

কচকচিয়া *Kuchkuchia.* A perennial. Bengal, (Serampore. Flower and fruit rainy season.

কচু *Kuchoo.* A perennial. Greece, Asia Minor, Syria, E. Indies. Flowers rainy season.

কঞ্জলতা *Kunja-Luta.* West-coast creeper. Large shrub and twining plant. Prome, Pagamew, Moluccas, Cochin-China, Bengal, (Serampore.) Patna, &c. Flower 8 lines, outside whitish, inside greenish, yellow-orange, delightfully fragrant, rainy and cold season.

কড়িলা *Kurila.* An undershrub. Both Peninsulas of India, Ceylon, Bengal, (Serampore.) Monghyr. Flower small, greenish-purple rainy and cold season; fruit cold season.

কণ্টকারী *Kanta-Karee.* A biennial. Bengal, (Serampore.) &c. Flower largish. bright-blue, and fruit whole year.

কদম *Kudum.* Large tree. Common about the villages in S. Concan, Bengal, (Serampore.) Sylhet, Patna, Gungachara. Flower small, orange-coloured, sweet-scented, hot season; fruit October and November.

কদু *Kadoo* লাউ *Laoo.* Bottle-Gourd. White Pumpkin. An annual and climber. Cultivated. Flower large, white, rainy and cold season; fruit cold season. The hard rind of the fruit used as a bottle for containing honey, &c. (Fukeer's bottles); a variety of it for making the stringed instrument, called Sitar; another variety as a buoy for swimming across rivers, transporting baggage, &c. (Royle. J. Grah.) The fruit of a wild variety তিতলাউ (*Tita-Laoo*), considered poisonous.

কথবেল *Kuthbel.* *Elephant or wood-apple.* Large tree, Moluccas, Coromandel, Bombay Presidency, especially at Guzerat, Bengal, (Serampore,) Assam. Flower small, greenish-white. anise-scented, March; fruit October. *Wood* hard, durable, From wounds in the bark exudes a very transparent gum, having the properties of Gum Arabic, and said to be better suited for mixing colours than it. The young leaves emit a fragrance of anise, and are therefore considered stomachic and carminative. The pulp of the fruit affords a very pleasant jelly, so closely resembling black currant jelly, as to be only distinguished by a slight degree of astringency. (*Wight*).

কনক চাপা *Kunuk-Chama.* A small tree. Both Peninsulas of India, Assam. Flower large, gold-coloured, fragrant, February and March; fruit May and June.

কনক চাম্পা *Kunuk-Champa.* Large tree. Peninsula of India. Assam. Flower large, white, fragrant, March, April and May; fruit cold season.

কনড়কা *Kanuraka.* An annual. Peninsula of India, Bengal, (Serampore). N. Doab, &c. Flower small bright-blue, and fruit, rainy season.

কমলা লেবু *Kumla-Neboo.* নারঙ্গী *Narungee.* Sweet-orange. A tree. Moluccas, Circars, Sylhet, Aurangabad, Khassya Mountains, &c. Flowers large, white, fragrant. In Honorable Company's Garden, flower February; fruit cold season. (*Roxb*). Here it has never fruited.

করঞ্জা *Kurunja.* A tree. Coromandel, common throughout the Concans, the Deccan, Amherst, Penang, Banks of the Saluen, Bengal, (Serampore.) Patna, Assam, Kheree-jungle, Deyra-Dhoon. Flower middle sized, bright-purple, hot season; fruit cold season. *Wood* light, white, firm, used for a variety of economical purposes. *Leaves* eaten by cattle. *Seeds* yield by expression a fixed oil, which is used externally in eruptive diseases.

করমচা *Kurumcha.* Large shrub. Moluccas, Both Peninsulas of India, Bengal, (Serampore.) Hindustan, Lower Kamaon. Flower middle-sized, pure white, inodorous, February, March and April; fruit July and August. Makes, on account of its strong sharp thorns, exceedingly strong fences. *Fruit* employed to make tarts, and preserves of various kinds, also pickles, and by most people reckoned superior for these uses, to every other fruit in the country, not even the mangoe excepted.

করলা *Kurula.* Annual and climber. Cultivated in all the warmer parts of Asia. Flower middle-sized, pale yellow, rainy and cold season; fruit cold season. *Fruit* bitter, wholesome, while unripe eaten in curry. It requires to be steeped in salt water, before it is cooked.

করাটিয়া যবানী *KuratiyaYuvanee.* An annual. Bengal, (Serampore.) Flower and fruit rainy season.

করেতা *Kureta.* An under shrub. Both Peninsulas of India, Bengal, (Serampore.) Flower smallish, yellow, rainy and cold season; fruit cold season. *Root* intensely bitter, and stomachic.

কর্পূর *Kurpoor.* Officinal camphor-tree. China, Japan. Flower small, pale greenish-yellow, March and April.

কর্পূর *Kurpoor.* An annual. Ceylon, Coromandel, Bombay, Bengal, (Serampore.) &c. Tropical N. Holland. Flowers 5 lines, greenish white, streaked with purple, rainy and cold season; fruit cold season. The plant has a grateful somewhat terebinthaceous smell, and a warm aromatic taste. (*Roxb.*)

কর্ম্মরঙ্গ *Kurmurunga.* Ripe fruit cooling, used in fevers.

কলকশান্দা *Kulkushunda.* Biennial and Perennial. Coromandel, Bombay, Tavoy. Bengal, (Serampore). Sylhet, Assam, Kheree-jungle, Deyrah-Dhoon. Flower small, yellow, rainy season; fruit cold season. Makes excellent hay.

কলমী লতা *Kulmee-Lata. Clove-scented creeper. Midnapore Creeper.* Shrub and Twining plant. The Concans, Guzerat, Bengal, (Serampore, Midnapore.) Flower large, pure white, expanding at sun set, and performing the air to a considerable distance with a fragrance resembling that of the finest cloves, rainy season; fruit cold season. Leaves used in curries.

কলমী শাক *Kulmee shak.* An annual. Coromandel. The Concans, Moluccus, China, Arabia, Bengal, (Serampore, Sylhet), Assam. Senegal. Flower large, pale rose-coloured, with a dark purple eye, rainy and cold season; fruit cold season. The tender top and leaves much esteemed and eaten.

কলম্ব *Kulumbo.* Perennial and Twining plant. Forests on the coast of Mozambique. Flower small, green, rainy season, much cultivated in the Mauritius. This plant produces the well known Calumba root, so much esteemed for its powerful antiseptic, tonic, and astringent properties.

কলসনড় *Kulusnur.* বরেথী *Burethee.* An annual. Bengal, (Serampore.) Flower rainy season; fruit cold season.

কলা *Kula.* Cultivated plantain.

কাওয়া *Kaoa. Coffee.* A small tree. Arabia Felix and Æthiopia, from whence it has been carried to nearly all parts of the world within the tropics. Flower large, pure white, sweet-scented, March, April and May; fruit November, December and January.

কাঁকুড় *Kankoor.* Hind. Kakni. An annual. Cultivated. Flower largish, yellow, hot and rainy season; fruit cold season. *Fruit,* when half-grown, pickled; when ripe, as large as an ostrich-egg, melonflavored, and, if hung up, keeping good for several months. *Seeds,* like those of other species of the Gourd-tribe containing much farinaceous matter, mixed with a large proportion of mild oil. The *meal* is an article of diet, and the oil is used for the lamp. Powder of the toasted seeds diuretic, and serviceable in promoting the passage of gravel. *(Roxb.)*

কাঁখরা *Kaukhra.* An annual. Mexico. Rio Janeiro. Java. Ceylon. Both Peninsulas of India. Bengal. (Serampore,) Hindoostan,

Lower Nepal. Flower small, deep blue, cold season; fruit hot season.

কাঁচ গড় গড় *Kunch-Gurgur. Job's Tears.* A perennial. Moluccas, Sunda Islands. Ceylon. Both Peninsulas of India. Bengal, (Serampore,) &c. Flower rainy season; fruit cold season.

কাঁটা গড়গড় *Canta-Gurgur.* A perennial. Circars. Bengal, (Serampore.) Flower rainy season; fruit cold season.

কাঁটা আলু *Kanta-Aloo.* A perennial and Twining plant. Bengal, (Serampore,) Monghyr, Morung, Vendalore, Sylhet, Kemaon. Not cultivated, though the root is large, white and reckoned very wholesome and palatable. Flower rainy season.

কাঁটা কচু *Kunta-Kuchoo.* A perennial. Cochin China, Penang, Singapore, Bengal, (Serampore,) Sylhet. Flower cold season; fruit hot season.

কাঁটা কুলিকা *Kanta-kulika.* Annual and Biennial. Both Peninsulas of India. Bengal, (Serampore.) Monghyr, Oude, Nepal. Flower 16 lines, pale blue, with the tube and throat, white ochraceous, rainy season; fruit cold season. Considered tonic, and diuretic.

কাঁটা গুড়কামাই *Kanta-Goor Kamaee.* A shrub. Peninsula of India, Bengal, (Serampore.) Flower small, white, hot season; fruit rainy season. An excellent hedge plant.

কাঁটা জাতি *Kanta-Jati.* A shrub. Arabia, Java, Ceylon, Both Peninsulas of India, Bengal, (Serampore,) Sylhet, Assam. Hurdwar, &c. Flower 1½ inch, bright orange, and fruit cold and hot season.

কাঁটা নটে *Kanta-Nuti.* An annual. Cochin China. Both Peninsulas of India, Bengal, (Serampore,) Assam. Flower, minute, green, rainy and cold season; fruit cold season.

কাঁটা মান *Kanta-man.* A perennial. Bengal, (Serampore.) Fruit cold season but rare.

কাঁটাল *Kantal. Jack-Fruit. Entire-leaved Bread-fruit.*—A tree. Moluccas, Both Peninsulas of India, Ceylon, Bengal, (Serampore.) Much cultivated. Flower very minute, greenish or (the male) white, crowded on a large receptacle, so as to form an amentum, January and February; fruit May, June and July. *Wood* hard approaching in appearance to Mahogany, much used for furniture. *Seeds*, when roasted, not inferior to the best chestnuts.

কাঁকড়া *Kankra.* A tree. Cochin-china, Moluccas, Java, Tenasserim, Penang, &c. Soonderbuns, Malabar. Flower largish, red. In Honorable Company's Garden. Flower hot season, fruit cold season. *Wood* hard, durable, yellowish.

কাক ডুমুর *Kaka doomoor.* A small tree. Coromandel, Hills east of Panwell, Kandella, Bengal, (Serampore.) Fruit receptacles in axillary pairs, peduncled, globular, umbilicated, hairy, the size of a large nutmeg, or on cauline racemes, appearing and ripening throughout the year.

This species is, from its being sown by birds, a great destroyer of houses and walls.

কাখড়া *Kakhura.* A perennial. Chittagong. Flower largish, deep-yellow, with a large white or pale straw-coloured, at the top bright crimson tuft, April; fruit none. The dry *root*, powdered and mixed with the powdered wood of Cæsalpinia Sappan, L. (*Bukkum*) makes the red powder, called *Abeer* or *Shagoo*, which is copiously thrown about during the Hooli, or Hindu holidays in the month of March. The root is also used medicinally.

কাগজী নেবু *Kagoojee-Neboo.* Long, small Lime. Bengal, (Serampore.)

কাঞ্চড়া *Kanchura.* কনড়কা *Kanouraka.* An annual. Peninsula of India, Bengal (Serampore.) N. Doab, &c. Flower small, bright-blue, and fruit rainy season.

কাঞ্চন *Kanchun.* Large shrub. Mauritius, Ceylon. Both Peninsulas of India. Bengal, (Serampore,) Assam. Flower large, pure white, and fruit whole year.

কাঠ গোলাপ *Kata-Golap.* A shrub. Forests of Nepal China. Flower largish, rose, half double, cold season; February and March; fruit hot season.

কাঠ শিম *Kat-Shim.* Biennial and Twining plant. Cochin China. Peninsula of India, Bengal, (Serampore,) &c. Flower large, rose purplish rainy season; fruit cold season, considered a poisonous plant.

কাঠ শোলা *Kat-Sola.* An annual. Bengal, (Serampore). Flower middle-sized, bright-yellow, purple-dotted, rainy season; fruit cold season.

কুকুর আলু *Kookoor-Aloo.* A perennial and Twining plant. Bengal, Calcutta, (Serampore.) Flower small, green, rainy season; fruit April. *Root* not esteemed, though eaten by the poor when hard pressed for food.

কুকুর চিতা *Kookur-Chita.* A tree. Peninsula of India, Bengal, (Serampore.) Assam, Tropical New Holland. Flower small, greenish-yellowish, May and June; fruit rainy season.

কুকুর চূড়া *Kookoor-Choora.* Large shrub. Coromandel Mahableshwur, Along the Ghauts, Hills at Salsette, Bengal, (Serampore,) Chittagong, Sylhet. Assam. Flower an inch, white, fragrant, April and May; fruit rainy season.

কুকুর জিহ্বা *Kookoor-Jihva.* A shrub. Both Peninsulas of India, Sirmore, Nepal, Lower Bengal, (Serampore.) Flower small pale-green, rainy season; fruit cold season.

কুচড়ি *Koochuri.* An annual. Bombay, Salsette, Kandalla Wurgaum, Bengal, (Serampore,) Rajmehal, Sylhet, Morung Himalayas. Flower large, beautifully blue, with gold-coloured anthers, rainy and cold season; fruit cold season.

কুচি কাঁটা *Koochee-kanta.* Shrub and climber. Peninsula of India, Bengal, (Serampore,) Sylhet, Assam, Deyra-Dhoon. Flower small, purple, gradually becoming whitish, hot season; fruit cold season.

কুচিলা *Koochila.* A tree. Martaban, Coromandel, Hilly parts of the Concan. Flower small, greenish-white, February; fruit none. *Wood* hard, durable, used for many purposes. It is exceedingly bitter, particularly that of the root, which is used to cure intermitting fevers, and the bites of venomous snakes. *Seeds* employed in the distillation of country spirits to render them more intoxicating. The pulp of the fruit seems perfectly innocent, as it is greedily eaten by many sorts of birds. Strychnine, an alcoholic extract of the seeds, has been found a powerful remedy in palsies.

কুচিলা লতা *Koochila-Luta.* Large shrub and climber. S. Concan, Coromandel, Khassya Mountains. Flower small, greenish-yellow. In Honorable Company's Garden flower April; fruit September, October and November.

কুদালিয়া *Koodaliya.* A perennial. Ceylon. Both Peninsulas.

of India, Bengal, (Serampore,) Monghyr, Nepal. Flower small, blue; and fruit whole year. The fresh plant bruised is sometimes applied to wounds that do not heal well.

কুন্দ *Koondo.* A shrub. Coromandel, S. Concan, Bengal, (Serampore,) Monghyr, Khassya Mountains, Assam. Deyra-Dhoon. Flower 18 lines, pure white, fragrant, rainy and cold season; fruit none.

কুন্দুরুমী *Koondoo-Roomee.* রুমী মস্তকি *Roomee-Mastuki Mastick-tree.* A small tree. S. Europe, N. Africa. Flower small, green. Produces the resin, usually called *Gum Mastick.* Has been introduced into Honorable Company's Garden.

কুমড়া *Koomra. Pumpkin. White Gourd.* Annual and climber. Cultivated. Flower large. yellow, rainy season; fruit cold season. The young unripe fruit universally eaten in curries.

কুমারিকা *Koomarika.* Large shrub and climber. Bengal, (Serampore,) Concans. Flower smallish, greenish, hot season; fruit cold season.

কুলগাছ *Kool-Gachh,* বয়র *Byur.* A small tree. Mollucca, Sunda Islands. Both Peninsulas of India, Bengal, (Serampore), Assam. The valleys of Gurhwal and Sirmore. Flower small, greenish-yellow, rainy season; fruit cold season. Fruit eatable.

কুলঞ্জন K*oolunjun.* A perennial. Sumatra, Moluccas, Cochin China, Singapore, Penang, Chittagong, S. Concan, Sylhet. Flower largish, pale-greenish, sometimes streaked with red, somewhat fragrant, April and May; fruit November. Yields the large Galangal root of the druggists. It has a faint aromatic smell, and strong pungent taste with some bitterness. In Cochin China it is found cultivated as well as wild, and the fresh roots are used to season fish, and for other economical purposes. (*Lour*).

কুলত্থ কলায় K*ooltho-kulay.* Annual and Twining plant. Coromandel, where it is chiefly found in a cultivated state, and called *Horse-gram plant.* Also cultivated in the Deccan and Bengal, (Serampore). Flower small, sulphur, and fruit cold season. *Seeds* grey. Produce about sisty-fold in a good soil and favourable season.

কুলিবেগুণ K*ooli-Begoon, Long Brinjal.* A perennial. Cultivated all over India. Flower largish, bright, bluish-purple, cold season; fruit hot season.

কুশ *Koosh.* A perennial. Peninsula of India, Bengal, (Serampore), Egypt, &c. Flower rainy season; fruit cold season. Used by the Brahmuns in their religious ceremonies.

কুষ্ট *Koosta.* কেউ *Keoo.* Perennial. Moluccas, Sunda Islands, Cochin China, Ava, Ceylon, Coromandel, Kennery Forests, Salsette. Throughout the hilly, wooded parts of the Concan. Bengal, (Serampore,) &c. Flower large, white, inodorous, rainy season; fruit September and October. The fresh roots are almost insipid.

কুসুম *Koosoom. Safflower.* An annual. India, from whence it has wandered into Egypt, the Levant, N. Africa, Europe, Madeira, &c. Flower large deep orange, cold season; fruit hot season. Cultivated in India for the use of the dyers, as also for the oil obtained from the seeds. *(Roxb).*

কৃপা *Kripa.* Large tree. Madagascar. Both Peninsulas of India, Banks of salt-water creeks in S. Concan, Sunderbuns. Flower small, white. Lately introduced. Wood strong, durable, used for posts and other parts of the houses, but chiefly fuel in Calcutta.

কৃষ্ণ কেলি *Krishno-keli.* A perennial. Peru. Domesticated in our gardens; flower and fruit whole year. Root purgative, whence the plant was formerly supposed to be the true Jalap-plant. Flowers large.

কৃ॰ চূড়া *Krishna-Choora.* Large shrub. Maluccas. Both Peninsulas of India, Bengal, (Serampore.) Flower large, sweetish-scented, and fruit whole year. Domesticated in the W. Indies.

কৃষ্ণ তিল *Krishna-til.* An annual. Flower deeper rose-coloured.

কৃষ্ণ তুলসী *Krishna-Tulsee.* An under shrub. Found cultivated about the Hindu temples. Flower small, pale-purple, and fruit nearly the whole year. Whole plant dark purple, and gratefully smelling. The juice expressed forms one of the ingredients of a celebrated and rather effectual nostrum for the cure of ringworms. *(Dr. Gibson).*

কেওড়া *Keora.* A small tree. Soonderbuns, Bombay &c. In Honorable Company's Garden flowers hot season. *(Roxb).*

কেয়া *Kea.* A shrub. Native place uncertain. Cultivated over all the warmer parts of Asia. Flower small, delightfully fragrant, rainy season; fruit cold season. The fusiform tough fibrous roots are used by basket-makers to tie their work with, and on account of their softness by the natives, as corks, (*Roxb*). Matting and package bags are made of them at the Mauritius. Avenues are formed of the shrubs themselves in China, Cochin China and Mauritius, and in the two former countries elephants are fed on them. (*Lour. Hardw.*) The lower yellow pulpy part of the drupe, is sometimes eaten by the poor during times of scarcity and famine, the same is the case with the white base of the leaves, which is consumed raw or boiled. (*Roxb.*)

কেয়া কাঁটা *Kea-kanta.* A shrub. Bengal, Calcutta. Serampore. Flower, small, almost as offensive as those of Sterculia foetida, L.; cold season; fruit rainy season; only employed for hedges. (Roxb.)

কেরালী *Keralee.* A perennial. Banks of rivulets, ponds, and wet places in Bengal, (Serampore.) Flower minute, and fruit rainy season.

কেলিকদম্ব *Keli-kudumba.* Large tree. Coromandel Mountains. Common throughout the Concans. Banks of the Irawaddi. Taong-Dong, Bengal, (Serampore.) Hurdwar, Deyra-Dhoon, Kheree Pass, Kemaon. Flower small, yellow, rainy season. Fruit April. *Wood* coloured like that of the Box-tree, but much lighter, and at the same time very close-grained. It answers well for furniture; exposed to wet, it soon decay's. (Roxb).

কেশরাজ *Kesho-Raj.* A perennial. Ceylon, Coromandel. The Concans, Bengal, (Serampore,) &c. Flower largish, bright-yellow, rainy and cold season; fruit hot season. The plant has a slight terebinthinaceous taste.

কেশরী মলঙ্গা *Keshuree-Mulunga.* An annual. Peninsula of India, Bengal, (Serampore.) Flower and fruit rainy season.

কানরাজ *Kano-raj.* A small tree. Bengal, (Serampore,) Kuvarikot, Islamnaghur, Oude, (Buch.) Assam. Nepal, Prome. Four petals white; the fifth somewhat sulphur within. Flower large, February, March and April; fruit cold season.

কানালা *Kanala.* শাদা হুড়হুড়িয়া *Shada Hoorhooria.* An annual W. Indies, Tropical America, Peninsula of India, Bengal, (Serampore,) Saharanpur, Nepal. Flower middle-sized, white, with crimson filaments and fruit nearly the whole year. Leaves eaten in curries; bruised and applied to the skin, they act as a rubefacient.

কান্দলি *Kandali.* An annual. Peninsula of India, Bengal,

(Serampore,) Sylhet, &c. Flower small, blue, and fruit rainy season.

কাপাস *Kapas.* Biennial and perennial. Molluccas. Both Peninsulas of India, Bengal, (Serampore,) Hindustan. Flower large, sulphur, with a dark blood-coloured eye, and fruit nearly the whole year.

কাফরি মরিচ *Kaphuri-Murich.* A shrub. Nepal. Cultivated all over India. Flower smallish, white, and fruit the whole year.

কামরাঙী নেবু Large, oval, smooth-skinned Lime. Bengal, (Serampore).

কামিনী *Kaminee.* A small tree. Monghyr. Foot of the Himalaya. Much cultivated. Flower middle-sized, white, strongly fragrant, hot and rainy season; fruit cold season.

কারণ ফল *Karun-phul.* A shrub, Calcutta, (Serampore) Flower small, greenish yellow, anise-scented, hot season; fruit rainy season. The leaves when bruised, have the fragrance of fresh anise seeds.

কলা *Kula.* Cultivated plantain.

কাল কচু *Kalo-kuchoo.* Leaves and petioles more or less purple-tinged. The roots never swell in the manner of the cultivated varieties, but send out numerous runners. The leaves and petioles are eaten by the poor.

কাল কর্পূর *Kalo-kurpoor.* An annual. Peninsula of India, Bengal, (Serampore.) Flower small, purple, rainy and cold season, fruit cold season. The whole plant is delightfully aromatic, and has a sweet pleasant taste.

কাল কস্তুরী *Kalo-kusturee. Musk-Mallow.* An annual. Moluccas, Java, both Peninsulas of India, Bengal, (Serampore,) extending northwards to the foot of the Himalayas. Flower large, sulphur, with a dark blood-coloured eye, rainy and cold season; fruit cold season. Abounds with mucilage, which in Upper India is used to clarify sugar. Seeds considered cordial and stomachic, used by the Arabs, mixed with coffee. (*Lindl.*)

কাল কালকাসুন্দা *Kalo-kalkasoonda.* An annual. Coromandel Mountains, Bengal, (Serampore,) Assam.

কালকাসুন্দা *Kalkasoonda.* An annual. Molluccas, Ceylon. Both Peninsulas of India, Bengal, (Serampore,) Assam, Nepal.

Flower-middle-sized, yellow, rainy and cold season ; fruit February and March. Smell of this plant heavy and disagreeable. Leaves eaten by the poor in their curries.

কাল কূঁচ *Kalo-koonch.* Seeds generally used by the jewellers as a weight. almost uniformly weighing exactly one grain, troy.—Root employed as a substitute for liquorice, being sweet and mucilaginous.

কালকেরা *Kalo-kera.* A shrub. Malabar, Bengal, (Serampore.) Flower largish, yellowish-white, cold season ; fruit rainy season.

কালজাম *Kalo-jam.* Large tree. Moluccas, Peninsula of India, Bengal, (Serampore,) Kemaon, &c. Flower small, white, March; fruit July and August. *Wood* hard, close-grained, durable. *Bark* strongly astringent, dyes excellent durable browns of various shades, according to the corrosive employed or the strength of the decoction. Fruit subacid, astringent, eatable. (*Roxb.*)

কালজিরা *Kalogira.* An annual. S. Europe, Asia Minor, Syria. Acclimated in the gardens of India. Domesticated about Serampore. Flower largish, white and fruit cold season. *Seeds* formerly used as pepper. It is esteemed as a condiment and stomachic.

কাল ঝাঁটী *Kalo-jhantee.* Large shrub. Common throughout the hilly parts of the Concan. Malabar Hill, Bombay, Mahableshwur, Sylhet, Hurdwar, Nepal. Flower 16 lines, indigo-coloured, with a whitish-yellow tube, February.

কাল দেবধান *Kalo-debdhan.* An annual. Cultivated in India. Flower cold season; fruit hot season. Grain much used for food.

কাল ধুতুরা *Kalo-dhootoora.* An annual. All over India. Flower very large, outside dark purple, inside whitish, and fruit whole year.

কাল মুগ *Kalo-moog. Black gram.* An annual. Native place unknown. Cultivated but not so much as the green gram. Flower largish, greenish-yellow, and fruit cold season.

কালমেঘ *Kalo-megh.* মহা তিতা *Maha-tita.* An annual. Java Peninsula of India, Ceylon, Bengal, (Serampore,) &c. Flower 6 lines, white, upper lip with each of the two side lobes marked with a dark purple streak and a couple of dark purple dots ; its middle lobe at base having a large purple spot on the inside, rainy and cold season ; fruit cold season, and February. Plant very bitter, and in the Peninsula of India much used in medicine. It forms the basis of the French *drogue amere.*

কাল শিম *Kalo-shim.* কাঠ শিম *Kat-shim.* Biennial and Twining plant. Cochin China, Peninsula of India, Bengal, (Serampore) &c. Flower large, rose purplish, rainy and cold season; fruit cold season. Considered a poisonous plant.

কাল হলদী *Kalo huldee.* কাল হলুদ *Kalo-hulood.* A perennial. Moluccas, Bengal, (Serampore.) Flower largish, red-yellow, with a crimsonish tuft, May; fruit none.

কালা *Kala.* A perennial. Bengal, (Serampore.) Flower 8 lines, deeper and lighter blue, with a white reddish tube, and a yellow stained throat, and fruit cold season.

কালী ঝাঁপ *Kalee-jhamp.* A perennial. Bengal, (Old walls about Serampore,) Peninsula of India. Nepal, Java, Philipines, Mexico, Brazil. Flower cold season.

কাশ *Kash.* A perennial. Arabia, Peninsula of India, Bengal, (Serampore,) &c. Flower rainy season; fruit cold season. Makes good mats for various purposes, and is used to thatch houses. Buffaloes are fed on this grass.

কুঁচ *Koonch.* Seeds red, with a black eye; flowers rose coloured.

কুঁদরু *Koonduroo.* A substance chiefly used as a grateful incense, but which also possesses stimulant, astringent, and diaphoretic properties. (Ainslie.)

কেশুরি *Keshoori.* An annual. N. and S. America, Egypt, Senegal, India, China, Moluccas, Java, Mauritius, &c. Flower small, white, and fruit the whole year.

কেশাড় *Keshar.* A perennial. Bengal, (Serampore,) &c. Flower and fruit rainy season.

কেশারাদাম *Keshara-dam.* Annual and creeper. Cochin China, Java. Both Peninsulas of India, Bengal, (Serampore,) &c. Flower largish, reddish-white, rainy season; fruit cold season.

কোক বরাদী *Koka-buradee.* ভুতুলশী *Bhoo-tulsee.* An annual. Tropical New Holland. China, Deyra-Dhoon, Oude, Hindustan, Sylhet, Cashmere, Bengal, (Serampore.) Flower minute, purple, and fruit cold season. Slightly aromatic.

কোক শিম *Kokshim.* An annual. Flower 4½ lines, bright sulphur coloured cold season; fruit hot season.

কোর্ণ নেবু *Korna-neboo.* A small tree. Garrow Hills. Foot

of the Himalaya, *&c.* Cultivated. Flowers white, tinged with red, fragrant, hot season; fruit rainy season.

কোদ *Koda.* মৈনা *Myna.* An annual. Bengal, (Serampore,) *&c.* Flower and fruit rainy season. Cultivated. The *Seed* is an article of diet with those men, who inhabit mountains and barren parts of the country. Boiled it is as palatable as rice.

কোদ *Koda.* An annual. Bengal, (Serampore,) *&c.* Flower and fruit rainy season. Cattle are very fond of both varieties, whether green or dry.

কোনী *Konee.* An annual. Peninsula of India. Bengal, (Serampore.) Flower and fruit cold season.

কোপি *Kopi.* *Cabbage.* A biennial. Eaten by all nation.

খএর গাছ *Khuera-ghach.* A tree. Coromandel. Hills about Vear, Salsette; and in some parts of the N. Concan, Yenangheun, Tavoy, Bengal, (Serampore,) Monghyr, Rajmahal, Morung Mountains, Assam, Delhi, Nepal. Flower small, white, hot and rainy season; fruit cold season. The old high-coloured wood, owing to the transference into it of astringent matter, is used for making the astringent extract known under the name of Catechu, formerly called Japan earth.

খড়ি *Khoree.* A perennial. Bengal, (Serampore.) Flower rainy season; fruit cold season.

খম আলু *Khum-aloo.* Perennial and twining plant. Wild in both Concans. Cultivated on the coast of Coromandel and in Bengal. Flower small, green, rainy season. Of yams it holds in Bengal the second place.

খরবজ *Khur-buj.* *Melon.* An annual. Persia, Kabul. Cultivated. Flower largish, yellow, and fruit hot season.

খসখস ঘাস *Khuskhus-ghas.* A perennial. Bengal, Peninsula of India, (Serampore). Flower rainy season; fruit cold season. The fragrant roots of this grass are well known all over India, and used for making tatties, covers for palankeens, large fans, &c. The grass is used for thatching bungalows in the Deccan.

খাজুর *Khajoor.* *Wild Date.* A tree. Common all over India. Flower March, fruit cold season. This tree yields, Palm-wine during the cold season. But free extraction destroys the appearance and fertility of the tree, the fruit of those that have been cut for drawing off the juice being very small. The mode of drawing off the juice is by removing the lower leaves and their sheaths, and cutting a notch into the pith of the tree near the top, whence it issues and is conducted by a small channel made of a bit of the Palmyra palm-leaf into a pot suspended to receive it. On the coast of Coromandel this Palm-juice is either drunk fresh from the tree, or boiled down into sugar, or fermented for distillation, when it gives out a large portion of ardent spirit, commonly called *Paria-aruk* on the coast of Coromandel. There as well as in Guzerat, and especially in Bengal, the Khajoor is the only tree whose sap is much employed for boiling down to sugar, mixed more or less with the juice of the sugar-cane. At the age of from 7-10 years, when the trunk of the trees will be about 4 feet high, they begin to yield juice, and continue productive for 20 or 25 years. It is extracted from November till February, during which period, each tree is reckoned to yield from 120 to 240 pints of juice, which averages 180 pints. Every 12 pints or pounds is boiled down to one of *Goor* or *Jagri*, and 4 of this yield one of good powder sugar, so that the average produce of each tree is about 7 or 8 pounds of sugar annually. This date sugar is not so much esteemed as cane-sugar, and sells for about one-fourth less. Baskets, boxes, mats and punkhas are made with the leaf-stalks.

খাজুর চড়ি *Khajoor-churi.* An annual. Peninsula of India, Bengal, (Serampore) Sylhet, *&c.* Tropical Africa, West Indies, Brazil. Flower large, deep orange-coloured, cold season; fruit hot season.

খামাচ *Khamach.* Annual and climber. Bengal, (Serampore.) Flower very large, white, rainy season; fruit cold season. By removing the exterior velvety skin of the large, fleshy, tender pods, they are, when dressed, a most excellent vegetable for the table, and the full grown beans are scarcely inferior to the large garden beans of Europe. (Roxb.)

খুদি ওকড়া *Khoodi-okra.* An annual. Peninsula of India. Bengal, (Serampore,) extending northwards to the banks of the Jumna. Flower small, greenish-white, cold season; fruit hot season. Cloth moistened with the juice of the green capsules, soon becomes blue on exposure to the open air. They, no doubt, contain colouring matter that might be usefully employed, probably similar to that of Croton tinctorium, L. (Roxb.)

খুদি জাম *Khoodi jam.* A small tree. S. Concan, Penang, Bengal, (Serampore,) Sylhet, Nepal. Flower minute, pale greenish, April and May; fruit July. Berries acidulous, of a pleasant taste.

খেত পাপড়া *Khet-papra.* An annual. Peninsula of India, Bengal, (Serampore.) Hindoosthan. Flower small, white, February; fruit hot season. Much used in medicine.

ক্ষেত পাপড়া *Khet-papra.* An annual. Ceylon. Both Peninsulas of India, Bengal, (Serampore) &c. Flower small, white, rainy season; fruit rainy and cold season.

খেসারী *Khesaree.* তেওড়া *Teora. Blue-flowered Chichling Vetch.* An annual. Spain. Cultivated in India. Domesticated about Serampore. Flower large, blue, and fruit cold season. Affords much wholesome green fodder, *Seeds* eaten.

গজ পিপ্পল *Guj-pippul.* A perennial. Paras. Bengal, (Midnapore, Serampore.) Calicut, Cochin China. On Chappedong. Moulmein, Rangoon. Monghyr Mountains. Flower rainy season; fruit January. At Midnapore it is cultivated for its fruit, which cut into transverse pieces and dried, is an article of some importance in the Hindu Materia Medica.

গঞ্জা *Gunja.* An annual. Siberia, Tauria, Scythia, Thracia, (Herod. 4. 74.) Whence the Hemp-plant was introduced into the West by the inhabitants of Marseilles; at least Hiero, the Syracusan, is said (Athen. 5. 40.) to have received it from the river Rhodus for ropes. Flower small, greenish white, and fruit the whole year. In India cultivated every where in the plains, near villages, for the sake of the intoxicating liquor called *bhang*, which is prepared from it, also for the leaves which are smoked to cause intoxication. "In the Himalayas it is indigenous, extremely abundant at elevations of 6-7000 feet, and of very luxuriant growth, rising sometimes to a height of ten and twelve feet. Here though it likewise affords an intoxicating drug, it is also known for the tenacity of its fibre, which is employed by the mountaineers in Ghurwal and Sirmore for making a coarse sack-cloth, and strong ropes for crossing their rivers." (Royle.) After so many experiments have been made to discover an efficient substitute for hemp, it is not a little remarkable that no attempts have been made to obtain the plant for commercial purposes, especially as its abundance and use in the North of India were fully known to Dr. Roxburgh, some years ago, and by him placed before the public. The grass-cloth of China would seem to be made of hemp, which the Malays use for sewing-thread and twine and for making fishing-nets. That the hemp plant is highly narcotic, producing giddiness, symptoms of incipient intoxication, rush of blood to the head, bleeding from the nose, strangury, aphrodisiacal sensations, &c. is well known. However, it appears, from Dr. O'Shaughnessy's experiments with the *churrus* or hemp-resin, that this substance is an efficient remedy against traumatic tetanus. (On the preparations of the Indian Hemp, or Gunjah, their effects on the animal system in health, and their utility in the treatment of tetanus, and other convulsive disorders. Calcutta, 1839.)

গরগোয়ালিয়া *Gur-goaliya.* Shrub and climber. Travancore, Permacoil. The Concans. Bengal, (Serampore.) Flower small, hot season; fruit rainy season.

গণিয়ারী *Guniaree.* Flower small, greenish-yellowish, unpleasantly smelling, rainy season; fruit cold season.

গন্ধন *Gundhun. Schallot.* A perennial. Syria, Asia Minor, Palestine. Cultivated in gardens. Flower small, white, with a green keel, cold season; fruit none.

গন্ধালী *Gundhalee.* গন্ধ ভাদালী *Gundho-bhadulee.* Shrub and climber. Moluccas. Both Peninsulas of India. Bengal, (Serampore,) Assam, Nepal, Japan. Flowers smallish, lilac-purple, like the whole plant, of a very offensive smell, cold season; fruit hot season. *Root* used as an emetic.

গন্ধ বেণা *Gundho-bena. Lemon-grass.* A perennial. Cultivated in gardens, but very seldom flowering. In the North of Bengal large tracts of waste land are covered with this grass. The fresh leaves are much used as a substitute for tea. The white succulent centre of the leaf-bearing culms is often put into curries, to give them an agreeable flavour. (*Roxb.*) The Natives of the Moluccas extract a pleasant tasted essential oil from the leaves. (*Carey.*)

গন্ধ ভাদালী *Gundho-bhadalee.* An annual. Both Peninsulas of India, Bengal, (Serampore,) &c. Flower small, white, and fruit rainy season.

গন্ধ মালতী *Gundho-malutee.* Flower 15 lines, pure-white, delightfully fragrant, rainy season; fruit none.

গন্ধ রস *Gundho-russ.* জগন্মদন *Jugan-mudan.* A shrub. Rangoon, Taong-Dong, Madura, Salsette, N. Concan, Bengal, Serampore.) Khassya Mountains, &c. Flower 7 lines, pale green ish-white, sparingly stained with purple, cold season; fruit February and March. Leaves and tender stalks have when rubbed a strong, not unpleasant smell. (Ainslie.)

গন্ধ রাজ *Gundha raj.* A shrub. China. Cultivated in Japan, the Moluccas, India, Cape of Good Hope, &c. Flower large, white, fragrant, hot season; fruit cold season.

গন্ধল রঞ্জন *Gundhal-rungan.* A small tree. Coromandel, Elephanta, Common on the Ghauts, and in the jungles about Nagpur, Bengal, (Serampore.) Flower 6 lines, pure white, very fragrant, March and April; fruit rainy season. Dák runners make torches of it.

গম্ভারী *Gumbharee.* Large tree. Coromandel, Neelgherry, Concans, Bombay Island, Prome, Trogla River, Saluen, Taong-Dong, Gorukpur, Sukanaghur, Oude, &c. Flower large, sulphur-coloured, slightly tinged with reddish on the outside of the tube, hot season; fruit cold season. *Timber* very strong and durable, resisting the influence of water and worms better than teak. The light wood of this tree is used for making the cylinders of the drums called Dholucks; also for making carriage pannels, as it combines lightness with strength.

গম *Gom.* Flower cold season, fruit February and March.

গয়াশ্বথ *Guyashwuth.* Fruit-receptacles axillary, sessile, paired, globular, smooth, the size of a cherry, appearing hot season; ripening rainy season.

গরাণ *Goran.* A shrub. Penang, Martaban, Tavoy, Soonderbuns. Flower small, greenish-white, hot season; fruit cold season.

গরাণিয়া আলু *Guraniya-aloo.* Perennial and twining plant. Only found in a cultivated state. Flower small, whitish, very fragrant, rainy season.

গরুড় *Guroor.* A perennial. Paras. Bengal, (Serampore.) Peninsula of India, Moluccas, New Holland, &c. Flower rainy season.

গলফিরিঙ্গী *Gulphiringee.* An undershrub. China, Cochin China, Common in gardens. Flower largish, rose-coloured, and fruit nearly throughout the year.

গাং বেনা *Gang-bena.* An annual. Bengal. Flower rainy season.

গাজুর *Gajur.* Flower cold season, fruit hot season. Forms a staple article of food in the eastern parts of the Deccan, during the cold season. (*Dr. Gibson.*)

গাদ বন্যা *Gado-bunya.* An annual. Peninsula of India, Bengal, (Serampore, but rarely.) Flower small, greenish-white, rainy and cold season; fruit cold season.

গাদা পূর্ণা *Gada-poorna.* Flower deep rose.

গাব *Gab.* A tree. Peninsula of India. Bengal, (Serampore,) Sylhet, Assam, Hurdwar, Deyra-Dhoon. Flower smallish, white, March and April; fruit rainy season. *Wood* of an indifferent quality, and not much used. Ripe fruit very astringent, rather unpalatable, eaten. Its viscid mucus is used for paying the bottoms of boats, and in Malabar, according to Rheede, for book-binding, both on account of its adhesiveness and its being obnoxious to worms. The unripe fruit contains a large proportion of tannin. An infusion is employed to steep fishing nets in, that they may be more durable.

গাব নল *Gab-nul.* A perennial. Bengal, (Serampore). Flower rainy and cold season; fruit cold season.

গার কলাই *Gar-kulay.* An annual. Japan, Moluccas, Nepal, Taong-Dong. Cultivated in gardens. Flower smallish, reddish-purple, and seeds black, cold season. Seeds in Japan commonly eaten in soups. (*G. Don.*)

গারুড় *Garoodoo.* মেরাডু *Meradoo.* A perennial. Peninsula of India, Bengal, (Serampore.) Flower small, greenish-white, with a tinge of rose, rainy season, fruit cold season.

গিমা *Gima.* An annual. Bengal, (Serampore,) Monghyr Himalayas. Flower small, January and February, fruit March The fresh, but especially the dried plant, is considerably bitter.

গিলা গাছ *Gila-gachh.* Shrub and climber. Lanowlee grove, near Candalla. Pretty common along the range of the Ghauts, Wanjura in Bamsari, Connatare, Moluccas, Penang, Moulmein. Banks of the Saluen, Sylhet, Assam, Nepal. Flower small, pale yellow, hot season; fruit cold season. *Seeds* used by the Ghaut-people as an antifebrile medicine (*Dr. Gibson*); by the natives in Nepal for washing their hair. (*Royle*).

গুগ্গুল *Googgul.* A small tree. Assam, Garrow-Hills. Flower small, reddish, February and March; fruit none. Produces the

Gum-Bdellium of commerce. and perhaps of Dioscorides. (*Royle.*) The whole plant, while growing, is considerably odoriferous, particularly when any part is broken or bruised, and diffuses to a considerable distance around a grateful fragrance, like that of the finest myrrh. (*Roxb.*)

গুড়দল শিম *Goordal-Shim.* Flower large, purplish. A larger variety. Cultivated.

গুড়ি শিওরা *Goori-shiora.* Shrub and climber. Coromandel, Malabar Hill, Bombay. The Ghauts, Bengal, (Serampore,) Sylhet Assam. Fruit-receptacles axillary, paired, peduncled, round turbinate, the size of a large goose-berry, scabrous, appearing and ripening the whole year. Bark of the root very bitter, given to remove pains in the bowels. (*Roxb.*)

গুয়া *Gooa. Betel-nut-palm.* A tree. Native place unknown. Commonly cultivated all over India. Flower small, white, fragrant, hot season ; fruit August and september. The Betel-nut is remarkable for its narcotic and intoxicating power. A kind of spurious Catechu is prepared from it. (*Ainslie*)

গুয়াবাবলা *Gooya Babula.* Large shrub. Flower small, yellow, fragrant, December and January ; fruit rainy season. *Wood* hard, tough, making excellent ship-knees and tent-pegs. Both Peninsulas of India, Bengal, (Serampore,) Scinde, Sylhet, Assam, Nepal.

গুরী *Gooree.* An annual. Bengal, (Serampore,) Peninsula of India. Flower and fruit rainy season.

গুলগা *Goolga.* A shrub. Moluccas, Soonderbuns, &c. Introduced into Honorable Company's Garden in 1810.

গুলদাউদী *Gool-daoodi.* চন্দ্রমল্লিকা *Chandra-mullika.* A perennial, China, Japan, Dindygul, Taong-Dong. Common in gardens. Flower middle-sized, or smallish, yellow, rainy and cold season ; fruit cold season.

গুলাচীন *Goola-cheen.* (Hind) গোবরিয়া-চাঁপা *Goburiya-champa.* A small tree. Cultivated in China, Cochin-China, India, the Moluccas, &c., where it is thoroughly domesticated. It is, however, no doubt, with the other Plumieras a native of S. America or the W. Indies. Flower large, reddish-yellowish-white, fragrant, especially during the night. Hot and rainy season ; fruit none, or very rare.

গুলাল তুলসী *Goolal tulsee.* An undershrub. Guinea, Penang,

Bengal, (Serampore,) Patna, &c. Flower smallish-white, rainy and cold season; fruit cold season. Whole plant very aromatic and fragrant.

গুলাসরফ *Goolasruph.* A shrub. Mountains of the Peninsula of India. Commonly cultivated in gardens. Flower large, gold-coloured, cold season; fruit hot season.

গুলঞ্চ *Goolancha.* Shrub and twining plant. Peninsula of India, Bengal, (Serampore,) Assam. Flower small, yellowish, hot and rainy season; fruit cold season. Used extensively in a variety of diseases by the Kaviraj's of India, especially in such as are attended by febrile symptoms not of a high inflammatory kind, and in fevers of debility. The parts used are the root, stems, and leaves, from which a decoction called *Pachuna* is prepared. A sort of extract called *Palo* is obtained from the stem, and considered an excellent remedy in urinary affections and gonorrhœa. From fifteen to thirty grains of the powdered root constitute a good emetic.

গেঁহুব *Gengwa.* A small tree. Moluccas, Sunderbuns. Salt Marshes at Bombay. Flower minute, greenish, hot season, fruit rainy season. The *juice* of this tree, and even its smoke when burnt, affects the eyes with intolerable pain, as has been experienced occasionally by sailors sent ashore to cut fuel, who, according to Rumphius and Roxburgh, having accidentally rubbed their eyes with the juice, became blinded, and ran about like distracted men, and some of them finally lost their sight. (*Lindl*),

গৈছি শিম *Gychhi-shim.* Flower red, pods 6-8 inches long; seeds black with a white eye.

গোয়ালিয়া লতা *Goaliya-luta.* Shrub and climber. Peninsula, of India, Bengal, (Serampore.) Flower small, red, rainy season, fruit cold season.

গোঁড়া নেবু *Gora-neboo.* Thick-skinned, small, oval Lime. Bengal, (Serampore.)

গোখুর *Gokhoor*, A perennial. Paghamew, Ceylon, Coromandel Deccan, Bengal, (Serampore,) Monghyr. Flower large, bright yellow, sweet-scented; fruit the whole year.

গোটি বেগুণ *Goto-begoon.* Large shrub. Bengal, (Serampore, &c.) Jamaica, Hispaniola, Bermuda Islands. Flower 8-9 lines, white, and fruit nearly the whole year.

গোথুবী *Gothoobee.* An annual. Bengal, (Serampore). Flower and fruit rainy season.

গোধ বেগুন *Godh-begoon. Love apple. Tomato.* An annual. S. America. Domesticated in India. Flower small, cream-coloured, cold season; fruit hot season.

গোবরা *Gobura.* An annual. Ceylon, Coromandel, Bombay, Bengal, (Serampore,) Nepal, &c. Flower middle-sized, reddish-purple, rainy and cold season; fruit cold season. The whole plant has a strong camphoraceous smell.

গোবরা নটি *Gobra-nuti.* An annual. Virginia. Bengal, (Serampore). Flower minute, greenish, and fruit rainy season. Cultivated

গোরক্ষ-চাকুল্যা *Gorukhya-chakoolya.* An undershrub. Both Peninsulas of India, Bengal, (Serampore,) Assam. Flower small, rose-coloured, rainy and cold season; fruit cold season.

গোড়ক্ষী *Gorkhee.* Flower small, white, and fruit whole year. Berries red.

গোলকাঁকড়া *Golkankra.* Perennial and climber. Bengal. (Serampore.) Flower large, cream-coloured, rainy season, fruit cold season.

গোলখয়রা *Gol-khyra.* A biennial. China. Flower very large, rose-coloured, February and March; fruit April. Is the origin of nearly twenty splendid varieties of border flowers. Leaves said to yield a colouring matter, resembling Indigo.

গোল মরিচ *Gol-murich. Black-pepper.* Undershrub and climber. Sumatra, Courtallum, &c. Introduced into Honorable Company's Garden, before 1793, but had not flower up to 1814.

গোল মলঙ্গা *Gol-molunga.* A perennial. Peninsula of India, Bengal, (Serampore.) Flower rainy season, fruit cold season.

গোল মেথি *Gol-methee.* A perennial. Bengal, (Serampore.) Flower and fruit rainy season.

গোলাব জাম *Golab jam. Rose-apple.* A tree. Both Peninsulas of India, Bengal, Sirmore. Cultivated. Flower large, greenish-white, February, fruit rainy season.

গোরী ফল *Gowree-phul.* A shrub. Neelgherries, Ceylon Khassya Mountains, Assam, Kemaon, Taong-Dong. Flower small, white, February and March.

ঘাস কচু *Ghas-kuchoo.* A perennial. Bengal, (Serampore.) Flower minute, rainy season.

ঘি নালিতা পাট *Ghee-nalita-pat.* An annual. China, Moluccas, both Peninsulas of India, Bengal, (Serampore,) extending up to Saharanpore. Flower small, yellow, rainy season; fruit September and October. Cultivated in China and Bengal.

ঘিমি শাক *Ghimi-shak.* An annual. Ceylon. Both Peninsulas of India. Bengal, (Serampore.) Flower small, white; and fruit the whole year.

ঘীনটি নটি *Gheenti-nutee.* An annual. Peninsula of India, Bengal, (Serampore.) Flower minute, green, and fruit rainy season.

ঘেচু *Ghechoo.* A perennial. S. China, Banks of the Irawaddi, Ceylon, Coromandel, Salsette, Concans, Bengal, (Serampore,) Sylhet, Monghyr. Flower small, purplish-white, with blue anthers, rainy season; fruit cold season. The roots are nearly as good as potatoes. Eaten by the poor.

ঘেট কচু *Ghet-kuchoo.* Perennial. New Holland, Cochin China. Both Peninsulas of India. Ceylon. Bengal, (Serampore,) &c. Flower minute, rainy season, the roots are exceedingly acrid, and used by the natives in poultices. (*Roxb.*)

ঘোড়া-মুগ *Ghora-moog.* Annual and climber. Bengal, (Serampore.) Flower largish, greenish-yellow, and fruit cold and hot season.

ঘোল-মহনী *Ghol-muhunee.* Undershrub and climber. Moluccas. Both Peninsulas of India, Begal, (Serampore, Monghyr.) Sylhet, Nepal, Saharunpore. Flower small, greenish, cold season; fruit hot season.

ঘৃত কুমারি *Ghrita-koomaree.* Much used in medicine.

চই *Chui.* Shrub and climber. Moluccas, Singapore, Penang. Introduced into Honorable Company's Garden in 1808, but had not flower up to 1814.

চনা *Chuna.* বুট কলায় *Boot Kalay. Chickpea. Chiches.* An annual. Spain, Italy, Levant. Cultivated in India. Flower middle sized, bluish-purple, and fruit cold season. Dr. Christie in *Madras Journal of Science, No. 13,* mentions that an acid, (oxalic acid) exudes from all parts of the plant, which is collected by the ryots, and used in their curries instead of vinegar. (*J. Grah.*)

চন্দন *Chundun. Sandal-wood.* A tree. China. Cochin-China. Both Peninsulas of India, Assam. Flower small, first straw-coloured, afterwards deep ferrugineous-purple, inodorous, and fruit nearly the whole year. Yields the Sandal wood of commerce, which is usually cut into billets, and disposed of in that state. It is burnt to perfume temples and dwelling houses, both in China and India. Reduced to powder, it enters into a composition for marking the forehead.

চন্দর মূলী *Chunder-mulee.* A perennial. Moluccas, Bengal, (Serampore.) Flower very small, greenish, rainy season; fruit cold season. *Roots* nutritious, eaten raw, boiled, or roasted.

চন্দ্র মূলা *Chundra-moola.* A perennial. Moluccas, Cochin-China. Both Peninsulas of India, Bengal. Much cultivated in gardens. Flower large, white, the lip at base marked with two dark-purple spots separated by a broad sulphur-coloured line, rainy season; fruit cold season. *Roots* fragrant, of a somewhat warm, bitterish, aromatic taste. Used both as a perfume and medicinally.

চন্দ্রা *Chundra.* ছোট চাঁদ *Chhoto-chand.* Large shrub in a rich soil, climber or twining plant, in a poor soil small and erect. Moluccas, Java, Cochin-China, Ceylon. Both Peninsulas of India, Bengal, (Serampore.) Hindoosthan, &c. Flower 8 lines, white, with the tube pale rose-lilac, the calyx red and the fruit shining black, throughout the year. *Root* used as a febrifuge, an alexipharmic, and to promote delivery in tedious cases.

চাঁপা *Champa.* A tree. Moluccas, Java. Cultivated in Bengal (Calcutta, Serampore.) &c. Flower large, deep-yellow, intensely fragrant, hot and rainy season; fruit cold season. Indeed, it flower and fruit nearly throughout the year. *Flowers* highly esteemed by us, especially for the use we make of them in our religious ceremonies.

চাঁপা নটি *Ohama-nuti.* Flower minute, greenish, and fruit rainy season. Peninsula of India, Bengal, (Serampore,) &c Cultivated all over the southern parts of Asia.

চাকন্দা *Chākunda.* Both Peninsulas of India, Ceylon, Moluccas, Bengal, (Serampore,) Assam, Senegambia.

চাকুল্যা *Chakoolya.* A perennial. Bengal, (Serampore,) Rangoon. Flower rainy season.

চাড় কচু *Char-kuchoo.* Disk of the leaves marked with dark-purple or bluish clouds, not cultivated. (*Roxb.*)

চামচিকী *Chamchikee.* Annual and Biennial. Coromandel, Bombay, Bengal, (Serampore,) Assam. Flower small, whitish, and fruit the whole year.

চামাটী পাটী *Chumatee-patee.* A perennial. Peninsula of India, Bengal, (Serampore.) Flower rainy season; fruit cold season. Very common on the banks of the Hooghly, where it helps much to bind and protect the banks.

চারিকোনা শিম *Chari-kona-shim. Goa Bean. Chevaux de Frize Bean.* Annual and twining plant. South America? Cultivated in India, and the Mauritius. In the latter place it is called *Pois carre.* Flower large, blue, cold season; fruit February and March. Pods used like French beans.

চালিতা *Chalita.* Large tree. Moluccas, Java, Ceylon, Peninsula of India, Bengal, Chittagong, Assam. Cultivated about Serampore. Flower very large, white, fragrant, July; fruit February. *Wood* hard, tough, used to make gun-stocks. (*Roxb*). *Leaflets of the calyx* agreeably acid; eaten either in curries, or used to make a sort of lemonade. *Leaves* hard, rough; and, like those of the other species, employed for polishing.

চিক্রাশি *Chikrasee.* Large tree. Chittagong, Cunnawady Hills, near Dindygul. Flower middle-sized, greenish-white. In Honorable Company's Garden flower hot season; fruit cold season. The *wood* of this tree, (*Chittagong Wood,*) is close-grained, light-coloured, elegantly veined, and employed by the cabinet-makers. (*Roxb.*)

চিচিঙ্গা *Chichinga. Snake-Gourd.* Annual and climber. Cultivated. Flower large, white, rainy season; fruit cold season. Fruit eaten by us.

চিড়িয়া ঘাস *Chiriya-Ghas.* A perennial. Bengal, (Serampore). Flower and fruit rainy season.

চিতা *Chita.* A shrub. Ceylon, Segaen, Prome, Penang, Rangoon, Courtallum, Malabar Hill, Bombay Hills throughout the Concans, Guzerat, Bengal, (Serampore,) Kutmandu. New Holland. Flower middle-sized, pure white, rainy and cold season; fruit hot season. The fresh bruised bark of the root is sometimes applied for raising blisters.

চিতুয়া বোড়া *Chitooah-bora.* A perennial. Paras. Bengal, (Serampore.) Flower rainy season.

চিত্র-চিড়ুয়া *Chitri-chirya.* An annual. Bengal, (Serampore,) &c. Flower and fruit rainy season.

চীন-ঘাস *Cheeno-ghas.* An annual. Cultivated in India. Flower rainy season ; fruit cold season.

চিনা-গোঁড়া-নেবু *Cheena-gora-neboo.* China, yellow-juiced Lime. Cultivated.

চিনা-নারঙ্গি *Cheena-narungee.* China. Cultivated in gardens. Flower middle-sized, white, fragrant, and fruit the whole year. Fruit very pleasant.

চিরতা *Chirata.* An annual. Mussooree, Nepal. Kemaon. Flower smallish, bright yellow. Has been introduced into Honorable Company's Garden. Flower ? In the garden here it has never succeeded.

চুঁচা *Chooncha.* An annual. W. Indies. Peninsula of India. Bengal, (Serampore,) &c. Flower and fruit rainy season.

চুক পালঙ্গ *Chook-palung.* *Country Sorrel.* Flower small. reddish, rainy season; fruit cold season. An annual. Africa. Cultivated in gardens all over Asia for culinary and medicinal purposes.

চুণ খড়কী *Choon-khurkee.* A perennial. Bengal, (Serampore.) Peninsula of India, &c. Flower cold season ; fruit hot season.

চুপড়ি আলু *Choopree-aloo.* Perennial and twining plant. Bengal, (Serampore,) cultivated. Flower small, white, rainy season. Most esteemed of all the yams among us, as well as Europeans.

চেঁচ্‌কা *Chenchka.* A perennial. Bengal, (Serampore,) Peninsula of India, Ceylon. Flower and fruit rainy season.

চেরুনটি *Cheroo-nuti.* An annual. Bengal, (Serampore.) Flower minute, greenish, and fruit cold season. Though not cultivated, used as a pot-herb, as it is considered very wholesome, especially for convalescents.

চেলাট পিপ্পল *Chelat-pipul.* মোম চীনা *Mom-cheena.* A tree. China. Domesticated about Serampore. Flower small, yellowish, March and April; fruit cold season. The Sebaceous produce of the *seeds* forms the vegetable tallow of China, which, however, is for the lamp, far inferior to Cocoa-nut oil.—*Roxb.*

চোর কাঁটা *Chor-kanta.* A perennial. Moluccas, Cochin-China, Sunda Islands, Ceylon. Both Peninsulas of India, Bengal, (Serampore,) &c. Flower rainy season; fruit Oct. and Nov.

ছাগল খুড়ি *Chhagul-khoori.* দোপাটী লতা *Dopatee-lata.* A perennial. Sandwich Islands, New Holland, S. America, Bourbon, Arabia, Mauritius, Ceylon, Moluccas, China. Both Peninsulas of India. Soonderbuns. Flower large, purplish rose-coloured, fruit nearly the whole year. Very useful on the sandy beaches, where it grows, in helping to bind the loose soil, and in time rendering it sufficiently stable to bear grass. Goats, horses and rabbits eat it. (*Roxb.*) The boiled leaves sometimes applied externally as an anodyne in cases of colic.

ছাগল নদি *Chhagul-nudi.* An annual. Peninsula of India, Bengal, (Serampore.) Flower small, purplish, cold season; fruit March. Whole plant inodorous.

ছাগল পটপটী *Chhagul-putputi.* An annual. Mauritius. Peninsula of India. Bengal, (Serampore.) Flower minute, greenish, cold season; fruit hot season.

ছাগল পাটী *Chhagul patee.* Large shrub and twining plant. Peninsula of India, Bengal, (Serampore.) Flower small, rust-coloured, rainy season; fruit cold season.

ছাগল বাঁটী *Chhagul-banti.* Undershrub and twining plant. Peninsula of India, Bengal, (Serampore,) Himalayas. Flower 6 lines pale green, internally tinged with purple, not unpleasantly smelling, (*very fœtid, Roxb.*) rainy and cold season; fruit cold and hot season.

ছাগল বাটী *Chhagul-bati.* Perennial and climber. Ceylon Both Peninsulas of India, Bengal, (Serampore,) &c. Flower middle-sized, yellowish, rainy season; fruit cold season.

ছাতিন *Chhatin.* Large tree. Moluccas, Coromandel, Hilly parts of the Concan. Vale of Saweetre, between Poladpore and the Ghauts. Bengal, (Serampore,) &c. Northwards as far as Mirzapore. Flower small, greenish-white, February; fruit cold season. *Bark* powerfully tonic, a rustic medicine in bowel complaints—(*Nimmo.*)

ছাগা *Chhya.* A biennial. Peninsula of India, Arabia Ceylon, Cochin-China, Bengal, (Serampore.) Flower small, white cold season; fruit hot season.

ছুঁচু মুড়মুড়ি *Chhoonchoo moormoori.* An annual. Bengal, (Serampore.) Flower and fruit rainy season.

ছোট আকন্দ *Chhoto-akundo.* An undershrub. Interior of Bengal. Flower largish, cold season; fruit none.

ছোট ওকড়া *Chhoto-okra.* ভুঁই ওকড়া *Bhooi-okra.* A perennial N. America, W. and E. Indies, Islands in the Pacific, New Holland. Flower minute, white, and fruit the whole year.

ছোট কট *Chhoto-kut.* A perennial. Peninsula of India. Bengal. (Serampore,) Nepal. Europe, N America. Flower 9 lines in diameter, pure-white, with a purplish base, February, March and April; fruit April and May.

ছোট কল্প *Chhoto-kulpa.* An annual. Both Peninsulas of India, Bengal, (Serampore,) Hindoosthan, N. India, Mauritius. Flower smallish, pale blue, and fruit nearly the whole year.

ছোট কিরাতা *Chhoto-kirata.* A perennial. Coromandel, Bengal, (Serampore,) Delhi. Flower small, yellow, rainy season; fruit cold season.

ছোট কেরই *Chhoto-keruee.* An annual. Coromandel, Bengal, (Serampore,) S. Europe. Flower minute, greenish-white, and fruit the whole year.

ছোট কোকসিম *Chhoto-kokshim.* An annual. Equatorial Africa, Java, Ceylon, Coromandel, Bombay Presidency, Bengal, (Serampore,) &c. Moluccas. Flower small, light purple, and fruit January, February and March.

ছোট গেঁদা *Chhoto-genda. French Marygold.* An annual. Mexico. Domesticated in India. Flower large, golden-brown, cold season; fruit hot season.

ছোট গোথুবী *Chhoto-gothoobee.* A perennial. Peninsula of India, Bengal, (Serampore.) Flower and fruit rainy season.

ছোট জাম *Chhoto-jam.* Large tree. Bengal, (Serampore,) &c, Flower small, white, March and April; fruit May and June.

Wood whitish, strong, close-grained, hard and durable. Fruit unpleasantly acid, astringent.

ছোট জাল গাঁটি *Chhoto-jalganti.* An annual. Bengal, (Serampore.) &c. Flower rainy season; fruit cold season.

ছোট ঝঞ্ঝন *Chhoto-jhunjhun.* An undershrub. Samulcottah. Prome, Bengal, (Serampore,) Monghyr. Flower small, yellow, rainy and cold season; fruit cold season.

ছোট ঝাঞ্জি *Chhoto-jhanjee.* An annual. Bengal, (Serampore,) Sylhet, Nepal. Flower small, yellow, with an orange-streaked scale, and fruit rainy season.

ছোট দুধিলতা *Chhoto-doodhee-luta.* Shrub and twining plant. Canton. Coromandel. Hills near Bagulcota and Badamee. South Mahratta Country, Bengal, (Serampore,) Sylhet, Assam, Nepal. Flower 2 lines, outside green, inside greenish-yellowish, with a white centre, rainy and cold season; fruit none.

ছোট নীলপদ্ম *Chhoto-nilpudma.* A perennial. Peninsula of India, Bengal, (Serampore,) &c. Flower smallish, blue, hot and rainy season; fruit rainy season.

ছোট পান চুলী *Chhoto-pun-chulee.* An annual. Peninsula of India, Bengal, (Serampore,) &c. Flower smallish, white, rainy and cold season; fruit cold season.

ছোট পিনে নটী *Chhoto-pine-nutee.* An annual. Peninsula of India, Bengal. (Serampore.) Flower rainy season.

ছোট ফুটিকা *Chhoto-phootika.* A shrub. Malabar, Travancore, Trincomali, Bengal. In Honorable Company's Garden, flower cold season.—(*Roxb.*)

ছোট বিচ তাড়কা *Chhoto-bich-taruka.* Shrub and twining plant. Chittagong. Calcutta, (Serampore,) Sylhet. Flower large, deep rose-coloured, rainy season; fruit cold season.

ছোট মটর *Chhoto-mutur.* *Grey Pea.* A small greenish variety of this much cultivated in Bengal.

ছোট মন্দা *Chhoto-munda.* *Parasitic.* A shrub. Bengal, (Serampore.) Flower small, greenish-orange, and fruit nearly the whole year.

ছোট মসূর *Chhoto-musoor.* *Hairy Tare.* An annual. Fields of Europe. Domesticated in Bengal and N. India. Flower small, pale-lilac, and fruit cold season. In the Upper Provinces used for fodder.

ছোট মেচেতা *Chhoto-mechheta.* An annual. Bengal, (Serampore) Sylhet, Assam, Oude, Banks of the Irawaddi. Flower small, pale blue, cold season; fruit hot season.

ছোট রক্ত কম্বল *Chhoto-rukto-kumbul.* A perennial. Bengal, (Serampore.) Flower large, rose-coloured, hot and rainy season; fruit rainy season.

ছোট লুনিয়া *Chhoto-looniya.* An annual. Peninsula of India, Bengal, (Serampore,) &c. Flower very small, yellow, and fruit the whole year.

ছোট শঁধি *Chhoto-sundhi.* A perennial. Bengal, (Serampore,) &c. Flower large, white, hot and rainy season, fruit rainy season. The *underground stems* (roots) especially of this, but also of the other species, are much sought after both as an article of food and medicine. The *capsules* and *seeds* are either pickled, or made up with curries, or ground and mixed with flour to make cakes.

ছোট সাদা মাখন সিম *Chhoto-sada-makhun-shim.* Cultivated,

ছোট হলকসা *Chhoto-hulkusa.* An annual. Mauritius, Bourbon. Java, Philippines, Peninsula of India, Bengal, (Serampore,) Himalayas. Flower small, white, rainy and cold season; fruit cold season. This plant possesses a considerable degree of peculiar fragrance. Its leaves are used as a potherb.

জঙ্গলী আদ্রক *Junglee-adruk.* A perennial. Rajmahal, Khassya Mountains. Flower large, pure-yellow, rainy season; fruit September and October. Bullocks sent into the jungles to graze in the rainy season in Northern India, have a portion of the roots of this plant given to them. (*Royle.*)

জঙ্গলী খাজুর *Junglee-khajoor.* A small tree. Behar. Flower cold season; fruit April and May. Fruit edible.

জঙ্গলী দাল *Junglee-dal.* An annual. Margins of tanks, lakes, &c. Bengal, (Serampore,) Peninsula of India. Flower rainy season; fruit cold season.

জঙ্গলী পাট *Junglee-pat.* বিল নালিতা *Bil-nalita.* An annual. Peninsula of India, Bengal, (Serampore,) extending up to the arid region on the western banks of the Jumna. Flower small, yellow, rainy and cold season; fruit cold season.

জঙ্গলী বাদাম *Junglee-badam.* Large tree. Moluccas. Both Peninsulas of India, Bengal. Flower middle sized, scarletishsulphur, very fetid, March; fruit rainy season. Seeds roasted, and eaten by the poor.

জঙ্গলী মটর *Junglee-mutur. Yellow Vetchling.* An annual. Corn-fields of Europe, Common in Bengal, (Serampore,) and near the banks of rivulets in N. India. Flower middle-sized, lemon coloured, and fruit cold season. Ripe *seeds* narcotic when eaten abundantly, but when young perfectly harmless.

জঙ্গলী হলদী *Junglee-huldee.* বন হলদী *Bun-huldee. Wild Turmeric.* A perennial. Presidency of Bombay. Throughout the Concans, Kennery forests, Parell Hill, &c. Bengal, (Calcutta, Serampore,) China, and various other parts of Asia, and the Asiatic Islands. Flower largish, aromatic, pale rose-coloured, with a yellow tinge along the middle of the lip, and the tuft large and rosy, hot season; fruit June. The *roots (round-zedoary* of the shops) are, fresh as well as dry, of a pale-yellow colour, and possess at all times an agreeable fragrant smell, and a warm, bitterish, aromatic taste. Used in medicine.

জটা কাঁকড়া *Juta-kanchura.* An annual. Peninsula of India, Bengal, (Serampore,) N. Doab &c. Flower small, bright-blue, and fruit rainy season.

জটা শালপানী *Juta-salpanee.* A shrub. Mauritius, Ceylon, Both Peninsulas of India, Bengal, (Serampore,) Assam, Kheree-Jungle, Deyra-Dhoon. Flower small, greenish sulphur, rainy and cold season; fruit cold season.

জডু পালঙ *Judoo-palung.* An undershrub. Coromandel. Bombay, Soonderbuns, New Holland. Flower very small, greenish, cold season; fruit hot season.

জবসা *Juvasa. Hebrew Manna plant.* An undershrub. Deserts of Egypt, Syria and Mesopotamia, Monghyr, Benares, Delhi, Common in Guzerat and S. Maharatta Country, Scinde. Flower smallish, red. Introduced into Honorable Company's Garden in 1810, but had not flower in 1814. Affords a grateful food for the Camel in desert places, (*Royle.*) The Hebrew Manna exudes from its leaves and branches. In the hot season, when almost all the smaller plants die, this sends forth leaves and flowers. (*Dr. Gibson.*)

জবা *Juva. Shoe-flower.* A small tree. China, Moluccas, interior of Hindoosthan. Flower large, crimsonish, nearly the whole year, fruit none. Petals astringent, used by the Chinese to blacken their shoes and eyebrows.

জয়ন্তী *Juyuntee.* A small tree. Ceylon. Both Peninsulas of India. Bengal, (Serampore,) Assam, Saharunpore. Flower middle-sized, rainy and cold season; fruit cold season. Cultivated and extensively used in the plain parts of the Deccan as a substitute for the bamboo. (*Dr. Gibson.*) *Wood* said to make the best charcoal for gunpowder. (*Roxb.*) *Leaves* used as a poultice to promote suppuration.

জয়পাল *Jypal. Hind. Jamalgota.* A small tree. Moluccas, Tavoy, Coromandel, Concans, Assam. Flower small, greenish yellow, hot season; fruit cold season. Produces the famous *Croton-oil.* The leaves have a very nauseous taste, and the whole tree smells offensively.

জরুদ কলমী *Jurud-kulmee.* Perennial and twining plant Both Peninsulas of India, Bengal, (Serampore,) &c. Flower largish, yellowish, with a dark purple eye, rainy and cold season; fruit hot season.

জল গড় গড় *Jul-gur-gur.* A perennial. Bengal, (Serampore.) Flower rainy season; fruit cold season.

জলপাই *Julpai.* A small tree. Assam, Khassya Mountains, Kamaon. Flower small, white. hot season; fruit rainy season. Fruit eaten in curries, or pickled. No oil can be extracted from them.

জল পাপড়া *Jul-papra.* An annual. China, Ceylon, Peninsula of India, Bengal, (Serampore.) Hindoosthan, Nepal, Chili. Flower small, white; and fruit the whole year.

জাতী *Jatee. Catalonian or Spanish Jasmine.* Shrub and climber. Common in gardens all over India. Flower 1¼ inch, white, externally suffused with purple, peculiarly fragrant, hot season; fruit none. The flowers are commonly used to make Durbar and Wedding garlands.

জাম্ব *Jumbo.* A tree. Moluccas. Cultivated. Flower large, greenish-white, hot and rainy season, fruit rainy season. *Fruit* somewhat aromatic.

জায়ফল *Juyphul.* The nut contains a volatile, as well as a fixed oil.

জারুল *Jarool.* Large tree. Circars, Courtallum, Valley of the Nagotnah river, near its source, Taong Dong, Tavoy, Amherst, Moulmein, Assam, Deyra Dhoon, China. Flower large, pale rose-coloured in the morning, at sunset purplish, hot season; fruit August and September. At Rangoon its *timber* is used to make knees for ships. (*Roxb.*)

জলগাঁটী *Jal-gantee.* An annual. Bengal, (Serampore,) &c. Flower rainy season; fruit cold season. Cattle very fond of this grass.

জলমুদী *Jalmootee.* An annual. Peninsula of India, Ava, Bengal, (Serampore.) &c. Flower and fruit rainy season.

জিওল *Jiol.* Large tree. Coromandel Mountains, Malabar Hill, Bombay, Elephanta. Pretty common on the Ghauts, Bengal, (Serampore,) Hindoosthan, northwards to the valleys of Deyra and Kyarda. Flower small, greenish yellowish, externally purplish, February and March; fruit September and October. *Wood* of old trees close-grained, of a deep reddish mahogany colour towards the centre. This coloured part is serviceable for many purposes, and looks well. From wounds in the bark issues a gum which, when dry, is like pieces of dry-glue. (*Roxb.*)

জীবন *Jeebun.* A small tree. Ceylon, Coromandel. Common along the foot of the Ghauts; Kennery forests, Salsette, &c. Bengal, (Serampore,) Sylhet, Assam, Nepal. Flower very small, green; and fruit the whole year. The inner *bark* of this tree, consisting of numerous reticulated fibres, forms a kind of natural cloth, used by the *Garos* for covering their nakedness. *Leaves* used by the Natives for polishing horn. (*Buch.*)

জীয়াশিম *Jeea shim.* Cultivated. Flower red.

জীলমরিচ *Jeel-murich.* An annual. Ceylon. Both Peninsulas of India, Bengal, (Serampore,) Hindoosthan. Flower very small, white; rainy and cold season; fruit cold season.

জুই *Jooi.* Large shrub. Peninsula of India, Tavoy, Banks of the Irawaddi, Bengal, (Serampore,) Monghyr, Nepal, Kemaon. Flower 11 lines, white, sweet-scented, March, and fruit rainy season.

জুঁই *Jooin.* Shrub and twining plant. Mauritius, Peninsula of India, Bengal, Assam, &c. Flower 1 inch, white, with a pale-greenish tube, very fragrant, hot and rainy season; fruit none.

জুঁইপানা *Jooin-pana.* A shrub. Rocky part of the Rotumda Ghaut, Mahableshwar. Common in gardens. Flower 1¼ inches, pure white, cold and hot season; fruit none.

জুপি কঙ্কা *Joopi-kunka.* An annual. Bengal, (Serampore.) Flower rainy season; fruit cold season.

জুম *Joom.* Large tree. Coromandel. The Ghauts. The hilly parts of the Concan, Bengal, (Serampore,) Assam, Deyra-Dhoon, Kyarda. Flowers smallish cream-coloured, March; fruit cold season. Fruit eaten raw or pickled.

জুয়ার *Jowar.* An annual. Arabia. Cultivated in India. Flower cold season; fruit hot season. Grain much used for food. The straw is reckoned very nourishing for cattle, and is a substitute for forage for horses, when grass is not obtainable. (*J. Grah.*)

জৈত্রী *Jytree, Albumen* (Nutmeg.)

যজ্ঞ ডুমুর *Juguya-doomoor.* Large tree. Coromandel. Common about Vear on Salsette, and generally by the banks of water-courses throughout the Concans. Table-land of Mahableshwar, Bengal, (Serampore.) Fruit-receptacles short-peduncled, turbinate, nearly as large as a common fig, downy, umbilicated, appearing and ripening throughout the year. The *fruit* disagreeable, eaten as a diet in diabetes.

যব *Juvo. Common Barley.* An annual. Native place unknown. Much cultivated in India. Flower cold season; fruit February and March.

ঝঞ্ঝনী আকরী *Jhunjhunee-ankuree. Common vetch.* Annual and biennial. Europe, Domesticated in Bengal, and Northern provinces of India. Flower middle-sized, bright purple, variegated with white-rose, cold season; fruit February and March.

ঝাউ *Jhaoo.* A tree. Coromandel, Banks of the Indus, Cutch and Scinde, where it is commonly used for fire-wood. Banks of the Jumna and Ganges. Flower very small, rose-coloured, rainy season; fruit cold season. The *ashes* of this tree, when it grows near the sea are remarkable for containing a quantity of sulphate of soda, and cannot be used as a ley for washing, as they coagulate the soap. When the tree grows in sweet soil in the interior, the ashes are free from the soda, (*Wight*). The galls of T. indica and dioeca are highly astringent, and are used both in medicine and dyeing. (*Royle.*)

ঝিঙ্গা *Jhinga.* Hind, *Torooi.* Annual and climber. Cultivated. Flower large, yellow, rainy and cold season; fruit cold season. The half-grown *fruit* is one of the best vegetables, and much used in curries.

টাকাপানা *Takupana.* An annual. Swimming on pools of stagnant water in the Moluccas Cochin China, Sunda Islands, Ceylon, both Peninsulas of India, Bengal. Flower small, pale-yellow, hot and rainy season; fruit rainy and cold season, (Serampore) &c. extending as far as Saharunpore. Tropical America. In Jamaica, in hot dry weather it impregnates the water with its acrid particles to such a degree, as to give rise to the bloody flux. (*Browne. hist. of Jam.* 330.) Cut into small pieces and mixed with rice, it is given to sucklings, who greedily devour this mixture. The leaves are almost tasteless, but their acridity soon attacks the mouth and lips as much as in Arum. (*Rumph.*) It is used as a poultice for the piles.

টানা জিনিয়া *Tanajiniya.* An annual. Bengal, (Serampore.) Flower rainy season; fruit cold season.

টিকৌওপড়া *Tikee-opra.* বিলপাট *Bil-pata.* A small tree. Peninsula of India, Bengal (Serampore), extending to the most northern parts of India. Flower small, deep rose-coloured, with a yellow centre, rainy and cold season; fruit cold season.

ঠাকরি কলায় *Takri-kulay.* Perennial and twining plant. Circars, Travancore, Bengal, (Serampore,) Prome, Nepal. Flower large, blue, rainy season; fruit cold season. Cattle eat the straw of this plant.

ডঙ্কানি *Dunkuni.* An annual. Both Peninsulas of India, Bengal, (Serampore,) Sylhet, Khassya Mountains, Himalayas, Flower middle-sized, white, rainy and cold season; fruit cold season.

ডাঙ্গা গড়গড় *Danga-gurgur.* A perennial. Circars, Bengal. (Serampore.) Flower rainy season; fruit cold season.

ডালিম *Dalim.* See আনার *Anar.*

ডুমুর *Doomoor.* *Common cultivated Fig-tree.* Small tree. S. Europe, N. Africa, Asia Minor. Cultivated in Arabia, Persia, and India. Fruit-receptacles solitary, sessile, turbinate, umbilicated, smooth, appearing March, April and May, ripening in June and July.

ডেঁফল *Dephul.* Bengal, (Serampore.) Not uncommon in gardens. Flower minute, internally rose-coloured; aments appearing in March, April and May; fruit rainy season. *Whole tree* and unripe fruit containing much tenacious, milky juice. The *roots* dye yellow. *Male spadix* acid, astringent, eaten in curries. Fruit eaten.

ঢাল কলমী *Dal-kulmee.* দুদিয়া কলমী *Doodiya-kulmee.* Perennial and twining plant. Both Peninsulas of India, Bengal, (Serampore,) Tirhoot, Assam, Nepal. Flower very large, white, fragrant, and fruit nearly the whole year.

ঢোল সমুদ্রিয়া *Dolsumoodriya.* A perennial. Bengal, (Serampore.) Both Concans. Towards the Ghauts. Flower small, white, rainy season; fruit cold season. *Root* astringent, mucilaginous. Reputed to be a remedy for the Guinea-worm.

তমাক *Tumak.* An annual. America. Cultivated all over the world. Flower large, rose-coloured, cold season; fruit hot season.

তমাল *Tumal.* Large tree. N. of Bengal, extending to Kheree jungle. Flower small, whitish, April and March, fruit none. *Wood* hard, black, heavy.

তরমুজ *Turmuz.* *Water-Melon.* An annual. Cultivated. Flower large, yellowish, January and February; fruit hot season.

তলদা বাঁশ *Tulda-bansh.* A tree. Bengal, (Serampore,) Flower May. The young thick shoots are, when about two feet high, tender and commonly used for pickle.

তাড় *Tara.* Large tree. Bengal, but scarce about Calcutta and Serampore. Flower March and April; fruit November and December. The *leaves* are employed to write on with pointed steel-bodkins, and also to tie the rafters of houses.

তাবা নেবু *Taba-neboo.* A large, globose, spongy-skinned Lime. Bengal.

তার *Taro* তারক *Turuko.* A perennial. Coromandel, South Concan, Æstuary of Irawaddi, Bengal, (Serampore,) Sylhet, Assam. Flower large, inodorous, beautifully rose-coloured, June and July; fruit October and November. *Root* considerably aromatic.

তারামণী *Taramuni.* A Shrub. China, Japan. Cultivated in Cochin China, India. Mauritius, West Indies, &c. Flower small, white, fœtid, cold season; fruit March.

তালগাছ *Tal-gachh.* *Palmyra-tree.* Large tree. Common in the Islands of the Indian Archipelago, as well as in the Peninsula and southern parts of India, whence it extends northwards along the Malabar Coast, and is described as almost the only tree seen on the flatter alluvium near the sea at Guzerat. It may also occasionally be seen as far north as 30°, or near Saharunpore. (Royle.) Flower hot season; fruit cold season. The sap of this Palm is abundant, mild, saccharine, and demulcent. It is collected by wounding the spathe, and drunk in its recent state as a refreshing beverage. The same is the case with the sap of Cocos nucifera, Arenga saccharifera, Caryota urens, Phœnix sylvestris, &c. The *fruit* is eaten, and considered very pleasant and refreshing. The *leaves* are employed for making punkhas. *Wood* very serviceable.

তালনরু *Talnuroo.* An annual. Soonderbuns. Flower and fruit rainy season.

তাল লুড়া *Tal-loora.* A perennial. Moluccas, Coromandel, Concans, Bengal, (Serampore,) Sylhet, Assam, Kemaon. Flower smallish, yellow; more or less throughout the year.

তালী *Talee.* Large tree. Ceylon, Moluccas. Introduced into Honorable Company's Garden in 1798, but had not flower up to 1814. In the Serampore garden it has been cultivated for more than 25 years without flower. This is the *Tali-pat*, or great *Fan-palm* of Ceylon, the leaves of which are used for thatching.

তিক চামা *Tik-chama.* A biennial. Coromandel, Bengal, (Serampore.) Flower largish, bright yellow, cold season; fruit hot season.

তিক বুমা *Tik-booma.* An annual. Bengal; (Serampore,) &c. Flower large, pale purple, February and March; fruit hot season.

তিক্তরাই *Tikta-rai.* A small tree. Travancore, Moulmein, Chappedong, Bengal, (Serampore.) Flower small, white, July and August; fruit hot season. From the seeds an oil is extracted which is used for many economical purposes.

তিক্ত শাক *Tikta-shak.* A tree. Both Peninsulas of India, Bengal, (Serampore,) Saharunpore. Flower large, white, becoming cream-coloured, with purple filaments, February and March; fruit rainy season.

তিত ধুন্দুল *Tito-dhoondool.* Hind. *Kerula.* Annual and climber. Peninsula of India, Bengal, (Serampore.) Flower large, yellow, rainy season; fruit cold season. Bitter in every part.

Fruit violently cathartic and emetic. *Seeds* in substance or infusion, used as an emeto-cathartic.

তিত কঙ্গা *Tito-kunga.* Large shrub and twining plant. Coromandel, Bombay, Elephanta. The ghauts, Mahableshwar, Bengal, (Serampore,) Sylhet, Morung, Assam. Flower smallish, green, inodorous, March, April, and May; fruit rainy season.

তিত পাট *Tita-pat.* An annual. Both Peninsulas of India, Bengal, (Serampore,) extending up to Saharunpore. Flower small, yellow, rainy season; fruit cold season.

তিত লাউ *Tita-laoo.* Annual and climber. Fruit of a wild variety, considered poisonous.

তিন্তুড়ী *Tin-tooree.* See আমলি *Amli.*

তিল *Til.* An annual. All over India. Cultivated in Egypt, S. America, W. Indies, the Levant, &c. Flower largish, white rose-coloured, hot season; fruit rainy season. *Leaves* emollient. *Seeds* contain a fixed oil, as tasteless as Olive oil.

তিলিয়াকরা *Tiliyakara.* Shrub and twining plant. Both Peninsulas of India, Bengal, (Serampore,) Oude, Assam. Flower small, cream-coloured, sweet-scented, hot and rainy season; fruit cold season.

তুত *Toot.* A small tree. Native place unknown. Extensively cultivated in Bengal to feed silk-worms. Flower small, greenish, February; fruit April.

তুন *Toon.* Large tree. Peninsula of India, Bengal, (Serampore.) Foot of the Himalayas. Flower small, whitish, honey-scented, May and June; fruit rainy season. *Wood* forms the Mahogany of India, though it is lighter and more loose-textured than Mahogany. *Bark* accounted febrifugal.

তুন তুনি নটি *Toon-tooni-nuti.* বন নটি *Bun-nuti.* An annual. Peninsula of India, Bengal, (Serampore.) Flower minute, greenish, and fruit rainy season.

তুলসী *Tulsee.* An undershrub. Common about the Hindoo temples; aromatic. Flower small, pale greenish rose-coloured, and fruit the whole year.

তেউড়ী *Teooree.* ত্রিবৃৎ *Trivrit.* A perennial. New Holland, Otaheite. Friendly and Marianne Islands, Ceylon. Both Peninsulas of India, Bengal, (Serampore.) Flower largish, white, with a tinge of cream-colour, rainy and cold season; fruit hot season. Bark of the *root* employed as a purgative. Cattle do not eat the plant.

তেকাটা সিজ *Tekata sij.* নাড়া সিজ *Nara-sij.* A shrub Coromandel, South Mahratta Country. Bengal, (Serampore,) Assam. Flower middle-sized, greenish yellow, cold season; fruit hot season. The inspissated milk juice of this species is said, in common with that of other succulent Euphorbias, to produce the drug Euphorbium. In India this is mixed with the oil expressed from the seeds of Sesamum indicum, and used externally in rheumatic affections, and internally in cases of obstinate constipation. (*Ainslie.*)

তেঙ্গ *Teng.* A perennial. Bengal, (Serampore.) Flower rainy season; fruit cold season. Culms used for screens and various other economical purposes.

তেপরিয়া *Tepuriya.* A perennial. Peru, Antilles. Much cultivated in India, N. Holland, &c., on account of its largish, yellowish, palatable berries, here generally called *Gooseberries* Flower small, yellowish, cold season; fruit hot season.

তেলাকুচা *Tela-koocha.* Perennial and climber. Both Peninsulas of India, Bengal, (Serampore), Saharunpore, Delhi. Flower large, white, and fruit the whole year. Ripe fruit eaten raw by the poor, and greedily devoured by birds; while green used in curries.

তেওড়া *Teora.* See খেসারী *Khesaree.*

তেলাঙ্গা চীনা *Telanga-cheena.* A small tree. China. Flower largish, rainy season. Fruit generally none.

ত্রিকাঁটা জাতী *Trikanta-jatee.* A shrub. S. Africa, Peninsula of India, Bengal, (Serampore.) Flower small, yellow, and fruit the whole year.

থলকুড়ী *Thulkuree.* Perennial and creeper. Asia, Africa, America. Flower small, purplish red, rainy and cold season; fruit cold season.

দইয়া খইয়া *Duiya-khuiya.* A biennial. Courtallum, Bombay, Bengal, (Serampore, Monghyr,) Lower Nepal. Flower minute, dark purple, rainy and cold season; fruit cold season.

দন্তী *Duntee.* হাকুই *Hakooi.* A shrub. Circars, Bengal, (Serampore,) extending northwards to the banks of the Jumna.

Flower small greenish-yellow, rainy and cold season; fruit cold season. Seeds esteemed as a good purgative.

দরমা *Durma.* নল *Nul.* A perennial. Peninsula of India, Bengal, (Serampore,) &c. Flower rainy and cold season; fruit cold season. The common *Durma-mats* are made of the stalks, split open.

দল *Dul.* An annual. Bengal, (Serampore,) &c. Flower rainy season; fruit cold season.

দশ বাহু *Dus bahoo.* A perennial. China, Japan, Cochin China, Nepal. Common in gardens. Flower 10-12 lines, below bright yellow, above dull-orange, with scarlet dots, scentless, rainy season; fruit cold season.

দাদমারি *Dad-mari.* An annual. Both Peninsulas of India, Bengal, (Serampore), Saharunpore. Flower minute, red, and fruit rainy season. The whole plant has a strong muriatic, not disagreeable smell. Its leaves, being extremely acrid, are used by the native practitioners of India to raise blisters in rheumatism, &c. Bruised and applied to the part intended to be blistered, they perform their office in half-an-hour, and most effectually. (*Ainslie.*)

দাদু মর্দ্দন *Dadoo-murdun.* Large shrub. W. Indies. Cultivated in India. Domesticated about Serampore. Flower large, orange yellow, heavy smelling, September and October; fruit February. The fresh leaves well rubbed into the parts affected once or twice a day, very frequently cure ringworms.

দানা *Dana.* An undershrub. China, Japan, Nepal. Cultivated in India. Flower very small, greenish, February and March; fruit hot season. *Leaves* of a slightly aromatic odour, and of a bitterish taste.

দানুরা *Danoora.* Small tree. Soonderbuns. Flower small, pale rose-coloured, hot season.

দাপু *Dapoo.* A perennial. Bengal, (Serampore,) Khassya Mountains, Oude, Nepal. Flower rainy season.

দাবীডুবী *Dabee-doobee.* An annual. Bengal, (Serampore,) S. Concan, Coromandel. Flower November and December; fruit January and February. "The natives of Bengal, esteem it a plant of great value, because they think it an easy, speedy, and certain cure for the troublesome eruption called ring-worms." (Hon'ble John Hyde in a letter to Roxb) "This accords with what Rheede, says of it, vol. 9, p. 139. Foliorum succus cum aceto mixtus impetigini resistit. Folia cum radice oleo incocta, contra lepram sumuntur." (*Roxb.*)

দামড়া শামা *Damra-shama.* An annual. Bengal, (Serampore.) Flower rainy season; fruit cold season. Several varieties of this grass are known to the Hindoo farmers. The *seed* is wholesome and nourishing, and constitutes an article of diet, particularly among the lower classes of the natives. It yields about fifty-fold in a good soil. Cattle are fond of it. (*Roxb.*)

দারচিনি গাছ *Dalchini-gachh.* A tree. Ceylon. Flower small, greenish-white, January and February; fruit May and June. *Cinnamon-tree.*

দুধ পিটলী শিম *Dood-pituli-shim.* Pods falcate. Flowers purple.

দুধ লতা *Doodh-luta.* Undershrub and climber. Coromandel, Bombay, Bengal, (Serampore,) Assam, &c. Flower 7½ lines, externally white, internally rose-coloured and purple-veined with a green tube, inodorous, rainy season; fruit cold season. Cattle eat it.

দুপহরিয়া *Doopahariya.* An annual. Both Peninsulas of India, Java, Moluccas, Bengal, (Serampore,) &c. Flower largish, scarlet, rainy season; fruit cold season.

দোপাটী লতা *Dopatee-luta.* See ছাগল খুড়ি *Chhagal-khuree.*

দূর্ব্বা *Doorbba.* A perennial. England, S. Europe, Caucasus, S. Africa, New Holland. Both Peninsulas of India, Bengal, (Serampore,) &c. Flower and fruit throughout the year. This most valuable grass forms three-fourths of the sole food of horses and cows in India.

দুলাল চাঁপা *Doolal-chumpa.* A perennial. Moluccas, Coromandel, Penang, Tavoy, Bengal, (Serampore,) Khassya Mountains, Assam, Nepal. Flower large, pure white, very fragrant, rainy season; fruit cold season.

দুলী চাঁপা *Doolee-chumpa.* A tree. Chittagong, Sylhet. Flower large, white, fragrant, April and May; fruit cold season.

দেতারা *Detara.* An annual. Bengal, Concans. Flower cold season; fruit hot season. Eaten by cattle.

দেব কাঞ্চন *Deva-kanchun.* Large tree. Mauritius, Coromandel Mountains, Banks of the Irawaddi, Martaban, Assam Oude, Kheree Pass. Flower very large, deep rose, cold season fruit hot season.

দেবদারী *Debdaree. Mast-tree.* Large tree. Java, Tanjore, Patna. Commonly cultivated about Calcutta and Serampore. Flower small, green, February and March; fruit rainy season. *Wood*, soft and useless.

দেবদারু *Debdaroo.* Large tree. Narainhetty, in Nepal, and at Simla, Bhotea pergunnahs of Kemaon. Flower August to October. Sometimes thirty feet in circumference. The *wood* is particularly valued for its durability, and is therefore much used in the construction of Himalayan houses, as are also the planks of Abies Pindrow. Deodar yields a somewhat coarse, very fluid kind of turpentine, which is much valued in Upper India as a stimulating application to foul and indolent ulcers. The leaves and small twigs of the Deodar are likewise brought down to the plains, being much used in native medicine. *(Royle.)*

দোমুটী *Domootee.* An annual. Ceylon, Tanjore, Banks of the Attran River. Bengal, (Serampore.) Flower large, white, variegated with red and yellow, rainy season; fruit cold season.

দোসরা শাক *Dosura-shak.* An annual. Both Peninsulas of India, Bengal, (Serampore). Flower small, greenish-red, rainy and cold season; fruit cold season. The tender shoots are eaten in curries.

ধনিচা *Dunicha.* An annual. Both Peninsulas of India, Bengal, (Serampore,) Gungachara, Saharunpore. Flower largish, yellow, purple-dotted, August and September; fruit November and December. Fibres of bark used for drag-ropes, and nets.

ধন্যা *Dhunya.* An annual. Greece, Levant, Tartary. Cultivated in India. Flower small, white, cold season; fruit hot season.

ধব *Dhub.* ধাইফুল *Dhaeephool.* A shrub. Peninsula of India, Bengal, (Serampore,) Oude, Deyra Dhoon, Timor, Java, China. Flower middle-sized, scarlet, with rose-coloured petals, February and March; fruit rainy season. Flower employed in India, mixed with Morinda, to dye red.

ধান *Dhan. Rice.* An annual. Cultivated. Flower rainy season; fruit cold season.

ধান লঙ্কা মরিচ *Dhan-lunka-murich. Cayenne-pepper-capsi-*

cum. A shrub. S. America? Flower smallish, white, and fruit the whole year.

ধুতুরা *Dhootoora.* An annual. All over India. Flower very large, white, and fruit the whole year. A strong narcotic. Sometimes fatally employed by thieves and other rogues, to deprive their victims of the power of resistance.

ধুন্দুল *Dhoondool, Hind. Porol.* Annual and climber. Cultivated all over India. Flower large, yellow, rainy and cold season; fruit cold season. Unripe fruit eaten by us.

ধুলি বাঁশ *Dhooli-bansh.* See বাঁশ *Bansh.* Large variety.

ধেনা *Dhena.* Shrub and climber. Mountains of Coromandel. Bengal, (Serampore.) Flower small, purplish-green, hot season; fruit rainy season.

ধেঁড়স *Dhenroos.* রাম তরাই *Ramturay.* A biennial. Peninsula of India, Bengal, in a cultivated state. Native place? Flower large, sulphur, with a dark-blood-coloured eye. Unripe fruit a favorite ingredient in soups, &c.

নড়দল *Nurdul.* An annual. Bengal, (Serampore). Flower rainy season; fruit cold season.

নড়ী *Nuree* নবাড়ী *Nabaree.* Small tree. Native place uncertain. Commonly cultivated in gardens. Flower small, reddish, hot season; fruit rainy and cold season. *Leaves* sudorific. *Fruit* succulent, sub-acid, cooling, wholesome, eaten raw, or made into pickles and preserves. *Seeds* cathartic.

নফটকী *Nuphutkee.* শিবঝুল *Shibjhool.* Annual and climber. All over India. Flower small, white, and fruit nearly the whole year. *Root* aperient.

নল *Nul.* See দরমা *Durma.*

নাগ কেশর *Nagkushur.* A tree. Cultivated in Bengal. Flower very large, fragrant, hot season; fruit cold season. Flowers found in the bazars in a dried state, being used in medicine, as well as esteemed for their fragrance. The grandees of Ava are said to stuff their pillows with the dried anthers of the flowers, on account of their fragrance. (*Roxb.*)

নাগদানা *Nagdana. Magwort.* A perennial. Europe, N. Africa, Levant, Siberia. Cultivated in gardens in India. Flower minute, purplish, February and March; fruit hot season.

নাগফুলী *Naga-phoolee.* An annual. Peninsula of India, Bengal, (Serampore.) Plains of North India. Flower small, white, rainy and cold season; fruit cold season.

নাগ ফেনা *Nag-phena. Hedge Prickly-Pear.* A shrub. S. America. Domesticated all over India. Flower large, (two inches in diameter,) bright yellow, and fruit throughout the year. "Upon this plant the Cochineal insects lately brought from America, thrive and multiply abundantly." *(Roxb.)*

নাগবলা *Nagbula.* নাগ বাড়্যালা *Nag baryala.* A shrub. Coromandel, Bengal. Flower small, white, rainy and cold season; fruit cold season.

নাগর মুথী *Nagur-moothee.* A perennial. Bengal, (Serampore.) Flower and fruit rainy season. *Roots* tuberous, aromatic, employed for perfuming the hair.

নাজুক *Najuk.* A perennial. Brazil. Cultivated in India. Flower small, purple, rainy season; fruit cold season. Commonly called *Sensitive plant,* the leaves falling on the slightest touch.

নাটা *Nata.* নাটা করঞ্জ *Nata-kurunja.* Large shrub and climber. Moluccas, Ceylon, Coromandel. Bombay, Ava, Bengal, (Serampore.) Assam. Flower largish, sulphur, rainy season; fruit cold season. One of the seeds of this plant pounded into a paste with three or four pepper-corns, and taken from three or four times a day in a decoction of Chiruta is an excellent febrifuge. The *seeds* are intensely bitter and powerfully tonic, and should not be neglected, at least, as an adjuvant, where *bark* and *quinine* disagree with the constitution. The whole plant is well adapted for hedges.

নামতি *Namuti.* An annual. Java, Peninsula of India, Bengal, (Serampore.) Flower small, yellow, cold season; fruit March.

নারঙ্গী *Narungee. Sweet orange.* See কমলানেবু *Kumla-neboo.*

নারিকেল *Narikel.* Large tree. Shores of equinoctial Asia and its islands, &c. Flower hot season; fruit cold season. The *root* is sometimes masticated instead of the Betel-nut. In Brazil baskets are made of the *small fibres.* The *hard case of the stem* is converted into drums, and used in the construction of huts. The lower part is so hard as to take a beautiful polish, when it resembles agate. The reticulated substance at base of the leaf is formed into cradles, and, as some say, into a coarse kind of cloth. The *unexpanded terminal bud* is a delicate article of food. The *leaves* furnish thatch for dwellings, and materials for fences, buckets, and baskets; they are used for writing on, and make excellent torches; potash in abundance is yielded by their ashes. The *midrib of the* leaf serves for oars. The *juice of the flower and stems* is replete with sugar, and is fermented into excellent wine, or distilled into *arrack*, or the sugary part is separated as Jagry. The tree is cultivated in many parts of the Indian islands, for the sake not only of the sap and *milk* it yields, but for the *kernel* of its fruit, used both as food and for culinary purposes, and as affording a large proportion of *oil* which is burned in lamps throughout India, and forms also a large article of export to Europe. The fibrous and uneatable rind of the fruit is not only used to polish furniture and to scour the floors of rooms, but is manufactured into a kind of cordage (*Koir*) which is nearly equal in strength to hemp, and which Roxburgh designates as the very best of all materials for cables, on account of its great elasticity and strength. The sap of this as well as of other palms is found to be the simplest and easiest remedy that can be employed for removing constipation in persons of delicato habit, especially European females. (*Ainslie. Roxb. Lindl.*)

নারিকেলী কুল *Narikelee-kool.* বড় বয়র *Buru-Byar.* Fruit eaten by all nation.

নাসা ভাগা *Nasa-bhaga.* An annual. Java. Both Peninsulas of India, Bengal, (Serampore,) Hindoosthan. Flower 6 lines, pale rose-coloured and white, cold season; fruit cold season and February and March.

নিম *Nim.* A tree. Ceylon, Peninsula of India, Ava, Bengal, (Serampore.) Hindustan, Assam. Flower small, white, honey-scented, February and March; fruit May and June. *Bark* used as a good substitute for Peruvian bark. *Leaves* especially mixed with equal parts of those of Vitex Negundo, L. are used successfully in various ways. The mixed, dried leaves, added to common poultices, act powerfully in preventing glandular tumors from coming to maturity. The same discutient effect is produced, after the application of leeches, in all kinds of bruises and sprains, by a watery or vinous infusion of them, particularly when spirit of camphor is now and then sprinkled over the cloth, steeped in the infusion. We have seen the greatest benefit from this application, in the worst cases of compound fracture. A *sacculus aromaticus* of these leaves, with a few grains of powdered camphor, seldom fail to afford relief in rheumatic affections of the ears, eyes, and teeth. From the *fruit* a bitter oil is expressed, which is used against worms, and. that, according to Dr. Buchanan, in doses of one ounce. This, Achil. Richard observes, is another instance, after the Olive, of the pericarp (pulp) yielding that substance which is usually obtained from the seed. The *seeds* after being skinned are used for killing insects, and the kernels, powdered and mixed with water, for washing the hair. *Timber* hard, durable, fit for ship-building—"Leaves beaten into a pulp, and thus externally applied, act, like a charm in removing the most intractable forms of psora, and other pustular eruptions." (*Wight.*)

নিমুকা *Nimooka.* A shrub and twining plant. Peninsula of India, Bengal, (Serampore,) Assam. Flower minute, greenish, rainy season.

নির্ম্মলী *Nirmmulee. Clearing Nut.* A tree. Coromandel. Hilly parts of the Concans. Adjunta Jungles. Banks of the Kalinadi River, South Mahratta Country. Hills about Parr. The Ghauts generally. Prome. Flower small, greenish-yellow, fragrant, April; fruit none. (*Roxb.*) In the garden here it has been more than twelve years without flower. The ripe *seeds* are dried and sold in every bazar to clear muddy water. One of the seeds is well rubbed for a minute or two round the inside of the vessel containing the water, generally an unglazed earthen one. In a very short time the impurities fall to the bottom, leaving the water clear, and perfectly wholesome. (*Roxb.*)

নিশিন্দা *Nishinda.* A small tree. Moluccas, Peninsula of India, Bengal, (Serampore,) Rajmahal, Deyra-Dhoon, &c. Flower smallish, odoriferous, beautifully blue, hot and rainy season; fruit cold season. A decoction of the aromatic *leaves* helps to form the warm bath for women after delivery. Bruised they are applied to the temples for the head-ache. Pillows stuffed with them are put under the head to remove a catarrh and the head-ache attending it. (*Roxb.*)

নীল *Neel. Common Indigo-plant.* An undershrub. Found wild at Quilon and in some parts of the Concan. Flower small, greenish-rose, rainy season; fruit cold season.

নিল অপরাজিতা *Neel-Uprajita.* Perennial and twining plant. Cuba, Arabia, Moluccas, Both Peninsulas of India, Bengal (Serampore,) Assam. Flower large, blue. and fruit whole year. *Root* and powdered *seed* purgative.

নীল কলমী *Neel-kulmee.* An annual. Found every where within the tropics, both in America, Africa, and Asia. Common in most parts of India, (Serampore.) Flower large pale blue, rainy season, fruit cold season. Seeds sold in the native druggist's shops, under the name of *Kala-dana,* as an effectual, quickly operating, and safe cathartic. Thirty to forty grains of the seeds, previously roasted gently, and powdered, make a sufficient dose for an adult. (*Roxb.*)

নীল ঝাঁজি *Neel-jhanjee.* Annual and twining plant. Peninsula of India, Bengal, (Serampore.) Flower small, pale blue, and fruit rainy season.

নীল লতা *Neel-luta.* Perennial and climber. Bengal, (Serampore,) Sylhet, Hindoosthan, Assam, Peninsula of India, &c. Flower very large, blue, with a white tube, and fruit the whole year.

নুণ বোড়া *Noonbora.* An undershrub. Peninsula of India, Bengal, (Serampore,) extending up the Gangetic Valley, nearly as far as Delhi. Flower small, rose-coloured; and fruit nearly throughout the year.

নুরিয়া *Nooriya.* Perennial and climber. Bengal, (Serampore, Monghyr,) Prome, Taong-Dong, Morung Mountains, Nepal, Kemaon. Flower minute, white, August, September and October; fruit cold season.

নোনা *Nona. Bullock's Heart.* A small tree. W. Indies. Domesticated in India. Flower largish, yellowish-green, of a vinous smell, hot season; fruit July—November.

নোয়া লতা *Noa-luta.* Shrub and climber. Coromandel Coast, Travancore, Jungly tracts of the Concan. Mawul districts. Shores of the Bay of Siam. Chittagong, Bengal, (Serampore,) Assam. Flower smallish, pale rose, fragrant, August; fruit cold season. Well adapted for covering trellises.

নৌকা *Nouka.* A perennial. Java, Coromandel, Concans, Bengal, (Serampore,) Tavoy, Sukanaghur, Monghyr, Nepal. Flower largish, bright-blue, rainy and cold season; fruit cold season.

পাঙ্ক শিম *Panch-shim.* A perennial. Pods straight; seeds reddish, flower white, large.

পটপটি চেঁচকা *Putputi-chenchka.* An annual. Bengal, (Serampore,) &c. Flower and fruit rainy season.

পদ্ম গুলঞ্চ *Pudmo-gooluncha.* Shrub and twining plant. Bengal, (Serampore.) Flower small, green, cold season; fruit hot season.

পরামূল *Puramool.* A perennial. Both Peninsulas of India, Bengal, (Serampore.) Flower 3¼ line, bluish-purple, inodorous, rainy and cold season; fruit cold season.

পরু *Puroo. Common Leek.* Perennial and biennial. Native country unknown. Cultivated in gardens. Flower small, greenish-white, or somewhat purplish, hot season.

পরুষ *Puroos.* A tree. Sunderbuns. Flower small, yellowish, rainy season; fruit hot season.

পলাশ *Pulash-Palasi.* Asiat. Res. 3, p. 469, and 4, p. 229. A venerable and holy tree; gave its name to the celebrated plain of "Plassey" in Bengal. A tree. Circars, Negapatam, Travancore. Common in the Concans, Kandesh and Goozerat, Bengal, (Serampore,) Chittagong. Sylhet, Khassya Mountains, Assam, Saharunpore. Flower very large, deep orange, February, March and April; fruit May and June. From fissures and wounds in the bark issues, during the hot season, a beautiful red juice, soon hardening into a ruby coloured, brittle, astringent *gum*; which, however, soon looses its colour by exposure to the air. *Seeds* considered anthelminthic. An infusion of the *flowers* of this and the next species dye cotton, previously prepared with alum, a bright yellow, which may be changed by an alkali into deep reddish-orange. (*Roxb.*)

পলু-বাঁশ *Puloo-bansh.* A tree. Smaller variety. Peninsula of India, Chittagong Mountains.

পাট *Pat.* An annual. Both Peninsulas of India, Bengal, (Serampore.) Flower small yellow, rainy season; fruit October and November used in India, and in Egypt, as a pot-herb. Cultivated in Bengal for the fibres of its bark, which are employed in making a coarse kind of cloth (*gunny* or *rice bags,*) cordage for agricultural purposes and boats, and Bengali paper.

পাটলি *Patulee.* পারুল *Parool.* A tree. Deccan, Bengal, Sukanaghur, Gorukpur, Kheree Jungle. Flower large, dark dull crimson, fragrant, hot season; fruit cold season.

পাটা শেয়ালা *Pata-seyala.* An annual. Coromandel. The Concans, Bengal, (Serampore,) Nepal. Flower small, white, rainy season; fruit cold season.

পাটী *Patee.* A perennial. Peninsula of India, Bengal. Flower rainy season, fruit cold season. Found in great abundance on the low banks of the Hooghly and rivulets near Calcutta, (Serampore,) &c. Where the tide rises high over it, it thrives most luxuriantly, and helps much to bind, and protect the banks from the rapidity of the water. (*Roxb.*)

পাটী খড়ি *Patee-khoree.* A perennial. Bengal, (Serampore.) Flower rainy season; fruit cold season. The natives make their pens of the culms of this and the next species, and use them also for screens and light fences. (*Roxb.*)

পাতর চুর *Pathur-choor.* A perennial. Common in gardens, Cochin China, the Moluccas, India, &c. Flower smallish, pale blue, very aromatic, April; fruit none. *Leaves*, and, indeed, all the parts of the plant, delightfully fragrant. The former are frequently eaten with bread and butter, or bruised and mixed with various articles of food, drink, or medicine. (*Roxb.*)

পাতি পাতি *Patee Patee.* মুক্তপাতী *Mookto-patee.* A perennial. Moluccas, Cochin China, Siam, New Hebrides, Coromandel, Bengal, Sylhet, Assam. Flower largish, pure white, hot season; fruit July and August.

পাতি নেবু *Pati-neboo.* Common, round Lime. Bengal, (Serampore.)

পান কাকরুল *Pankakrool.* A perennial. Bengal, (Serampore.) Flower rainy season.

পানতোরাশি *Pantorasee.* A perennial. Bengal. Flower small, white, cold and hot season; fruit hot season. *Leaves* and *seeds* somewhat unpleasantly aromatic. Not used by us.

পান মহুরি *Pan-muhoree.* An annual. Native place? Cultivated in Bengal. Flower small, bright-yellow, February; fruit March and April. *Seeds* of a pleasant, sweet, warmish taste, used for culinary and medicinal purposes.

পান সিউলি *Pan-shiooli.* Shrub and climber. Coromandel, Concans, Bengal, (Serampore.) Flower small, greenish-white; and fruit the whole year.

পান *Pan.* *Betel-leaf.* Shrub and climber or creeping. Native place unknown. Cultivated all over India. *Aments* appearing rainy and cold season.

পানা *Pana.* An annual. Bengal. In Honorable Company's Garden flower rainy season.

পানিয়ালা *Paneeyala.* A tree. Assam, Monghyr, Nepal. Flower minute, greenish, cold season. *Fruit* palatable, reckoned wholesome.

পানি কলা *Panee-kula.* An annual. Sunda Islands, Ceylon, Coromandel, Bombay. The Concans, Melloon, Bengal, (Serampore.) Sylhet, Assam, Nepal, Egypt. Flower 1-2 inches in diameter, whitish, fugacious, longitudinally veined, rainy season; fruit cold season.

পানি কাঞ্চড়া *Panee-kanchura.* An annual. Coromandel. Bengal, (Serampore.) Flower smallish, deep azure, and fruit rainy season.

পানি জমা *Panee-juma.* A small tree. Kheree Pass, along the foot of the Mountains, and in other hot parts of India, as Bengal and the Peninsula. In the Presidency of Bombay, the vale of Yena, and other moist places, Mahableshwar; various places of the Southern Mahratta Country. Flower hot and rainy season.

পানি দূর্ব্বা *Panee-doorba.* A perennial. Peninsula of India. Bengal, (Serampore.) W. Indies. Flower rainy season; fruit cold season.

পানি নাজুক *Panee-najuk.* An annual. Tanks in both the Peninsulas of India. Cochin-China. Bengal, (Serampore,) Sylhet Assam. Flower small, reddish, rainy and cold season; fruit cold season.

পানি ফল *Panee-phul.* সিঙ্গারা *Singara.* An annual. Both Peninsulas of India, Bengal, (Serampore,) Nepal. Flower smallish, white, May and June; fruit cold season. *Fruit* sold in the bazar, and eaten by us. In Guzerat it forms an important article of food. During the *Hooly* festival a red dye is made of it mixed with a yellow dye procured from the flowers of Butea frondosa.

পানি মরিচ *Panee-murich.* An annual. Bengal, (Serampore.) Flower small, white, rainy season; fruit cold season.

পানি মলঙ্গা *Panee-mulunga.* A perennial. Peninsula of India. Bengal, (Serampore.) St. Cruz. Benin. Flower and fruit rainy season.

পানি শিড়া *Panee-shira.* Perennial and climber. Borders of tanks, &c. in Bengal and the Peninsula of India.

পানি সাড়া *Panee-Sara.* A shrub. Bengal, (Serampore.) Flower middle-sized, white, rainy season; fruit cold season. Often employed with Trophis aspera, Retz. for making hedges.

পানি লতা *Panee-luta.* Shrub and climber. Both Peninsulas of India, Bengal, Soonderbuns, (Serampore.) Flower middle sized, pale rose-coloured. April and May; fruit rainy season.

পালক জুই *Paluka-jooi.* A small tree. Bengal, (Serampore.) Monghyr. Flower 5 lines, pure white, sweet-scented, March and April; fruit June and July.

পালঙ্গ শাক *Palung-shak.* An annual. Native place unknown. Commonly cultivated in Bengal and the N. Circars. Flower small, green, and fruit cold season. *Leaves* (only) used in curries.

পালিতা মান্দার *Palita-mundar.* A tree. Coromandel. Common throughout the Concans. Amherst, Martaban, Bengal, (Serampore.) Assam. Flower large, greenish dark purple scarlet, February and March; fruit June and July. *Wood* light and soft, much used by toy-makers; also generally employed for constructing Catamarans (*Wight.*) The tree is used to support the black pepper vine, to protect young coffee trees, &c.

পিপুল *Pipool.* *Long-pepper.* Shrub and creeper. Banks of water-courses towards the Circar Mountains. S. Concan. Banks of the Irawaddi, Bengal, (Serampore.) Sylhet. Aments appearing rainy season; fruit cold season.

পিঙ্গি নাছি. *Pingi-nachhi.* An annual. Bengal, (Serampore,) &c. Flower rainy season; fruit cold season.

পিটলি *Pitulee.* A tree. Coromandel. Parell Hill. Bombay. Common in the jungle between Nagotnah and the Pass leading to Judapore. Bengal, (Serampore.) Flower small, whitish-greenish, hot season; fruit rainy season. *Wood* soft and of little value.

পিড়িঙ্গ *Piring.* An annual. S. France. Cultivated in India. Flower small, yellow; and fruit cold season.

পিনিস *Pinish.* An annual. Much cultivated in Bengal. Native place uncertain. Flower very small, green, cold season; fruit hot season. This pot-herb is much esteemed by us.

পিপিরি সারা *Pipiri-sara.* A perennial. Flower very small,

greenish, rainy season, fruit cold season, Bengal, (Scrampore,) Nepal, Assam, Java.

পিপ্পল *Pippul.* A tree. Common all over India. Fruit-receptacles axillary, paired, sessile, depressed, the size of a small cherry, appearing hot season, ripening raihy season. Birds are very fond of the fruit, eat it greedily, and often drop the seeds in cracks of buildings, where they vegetate, occasioning great damage if not removed in time. *Wood* light and of little use.

পীয়া-বাঁস *Peea-bansh.* A larger variety used chiefly for scaffolding and building the better and larger sorts of houses. It differs from *Tulda-bansh* by its greater length and thickness of the joints.

পিয়াশাল *Piyashal.* See আশান *Ashan.*

পির আলু *Pir-aloo.* A small tree. Coromandel. Banks of rivers in the Concan. South Mahratta Country. Ataveesy, where the coolies roast and eat the fruit. Bengal, (Serampore.) Deyra Dhoon, Kheree Pass. Flower large, white, fragrant, hot season; fruit cold season.

পীত শাল *Peet-sal.* A tree. Columala. Neelgherries. Common in some parts of the Concans, Rajpeepla jungles. Assam. Flower smallish, white, tinged with yellow, rainy season; fruit hot season. *Wood* reddish, employed for making doors, window frames, &c. *Bark* and *leaves* afford gum *Kino*, exported in considerable quantities from Malabar. (*Dr. Gibson.*) Long ago Dr. Rosburgh had said, "The specimen of the *gum Kino Tree.* in the Banksian Herbarium, is perfectly like P. Marsupium."

পিপুলী ঝঞ্ঝন *Peepooli-jhunjhun.* An annual. Peninsula of India. Bengal, (Serampore,) Assam, Deyra-Dhoon, Kheree Jungle. Flower large, bright yellow, rainy and cold season: fruit cold season.

পুঁখা *Punkha.* An annual. Peninsula of India, Bengal, (Serampore,) Monghyr. Flower minute, white, rainy season; fruit rainy and cold season.

পুদিনা *Poodina.* A perennial. Temperate parts of Europe. Cape of Good Hope. N. and S. America, where, it is probably but domesticated. Flower small, purplish. Does not flower in Lower Bengal. It was introduced into Honorable Company's Garden in 1795, but had not flower up to 1814.

পুন্নাগ *Poonnag.* A tree. Coromandel, Parell Hill, Bombay. Hills throughout the Concans. Common in the jungles between Mundighur and Sanklee, Assam. Has not flower here, nor had it done so in Honorable Company's Garden in 1814, though introduced in 1797. The red, mealy powder which covers the capsules is used to dye scarlet.

পুন্নাগ চাঁপা *Poonnag-champa.* A perennial. Banks of the Saluen. Sylhet. Coromandel. Flower large, more or less rose-coloured, with the lip orange yellow on a dark crimson ground, April and May ; fruit September and October.

পুঁই শাক *Pooin-shak.* Perennial and twining plant. Flower small, rose-coloured, January, February and March ; fruit hot season. A native of most parts of India, and much cultivated as a pot-herb.

পেঁপিয়া *Pepiya.* A tree. S. America. Domesticated in India. Flower middle-sized, pale yellow, fragrant ; and fruit nearly the whole year. Trees either straight and without branches like a palm, or branched. *Leaves* employed by the negroes in the W. Indies to wash their linen, instead of soap. *Fruit,* when unripe, used in curries, also pickled, and made into a preserve ; when ripe, the soft, yellow pulp, which is very delicious to many, is eaten without the addition of pepper and sugar, as in the W. Indies. It is certainly wholesome, more especially when some of the olive-coloured, pungent, caper-like seeds are partaken of at the same time. *Juice of the pulp* employed in the W. Indies against freckles, *of the unripe fruit* as an efficient vermifuge. "The tree has, moreover, the singular property of rendering the toughest animal substances tender, by causing a separation of the muscular fibre ; its very vapour even does this ; newly-killed meat suspended among the leaves, and even old hogs and old poultry, when fed on the leaves and fruit, become tender in a few hours. A principal constituent of the juice of the unripe fruit is fibrine, a principle otherwise supposed peculiar to the animal kingdom and to fungi." (*Lindl.*)

পেয়াজ *Peyaj.* A biennial. *Common Onion.* Native country unknown. Commonly cultivated. Flower small, white, or greenish-purplish-white with a green keel, cold season ; fruit none.

পেটারি *Petaree.* A biennial. Peninsula of India, Bengal, (Serampore.) Flower largish, orange, rainy and cold season ; fruit cold season.

পেটিনড় *Petinur.* An annual. Bengal, (Serampore,) &c. Flower rainy season; fruit cold season.

পেয়ারা *Peyara.* A small tree. West Indies, Tropical S. America. Domesticated in India. Flower largish, white, sweetish scented, hot season; fruit rainy season.

পোরেশ *Poresh.* A tree. Society Islands, Guinea, Courtallum, Singapore, Bengal. Flower large, sulphur, with a dark blood-coloured eye, rainy season; fruit cold season. *Wood* used for making rollers, and other purposes, where closeness of grain is required. The *fruit* abounds in a yellow pigment, which might perhaps be turned to some account.

পোরেশ পিপ্পল *Poresh-pippul.* A tree. Coromandel, Bengal. Flower rainy and cold season, fruit cold season.

পোস্ত *Posto.* Extensively cultivated in India. The *juice* expressed from the seeds, held to be very useful in chronic diarrhœa. Their *oil* pure, sweet, for culinary purposes almost as good as olive oil.

ফলসা *Phulsa.* A small tree. Peninsula of India. Bengal, (Serampore.) Flower middle-sized, yellowish-orange, cold season; fruit hot season. *Berries* acid, palatable.

ফিরকি টগর *Phirki-tugur.* A shrub. Moluccas, Manilla, Ceylon. Both Peninsulas of India, Bengal, (Serampore,) Sylhet, Nepal. Flower 2 inches, pure white, fragrant, the tube bright yellow within, hot and rainy season; fruit cold season.

ফুটী *Phootee.* An annual. Cultivated. Flower largish, yellow, February; fruit hot season. *Fruit* much eaten; when young, a good substitute for the common cucumber; when ripe, (after bursting spontaneously) with a little sugar little inferior to the melon, and reckoned very wholesome. *Seed* now and then ground into a kind of meal.

ফুল কোপি *Phool-kopi. Cauliflower.* A biennial. Europe. Cultivated in India.

ফুল সোলা *Phool-sola.* A perennial. Coromandal, Bengal, (Serampore,) Sylhet, Assam, Saharunpore. Flower middle-sized, brownish orange, rainy season; fruit cold season. The larger plants are particularly light, white, and spongy. They are gathered during April and May, and converted into a great variety of toys, floats for fishing nets, gentlemen's hats &c.

বক *Buko.* A tree. Moluccas. Both Peninsulas of India, Bengal, (Serampore,) Assam. Flower large, nearly the whole year; fruit cold season. Employed for training the betelplant. *Wood* only fit for fuel. Tender *leaves, flowers* and young *legumes* much eaten; the young *shoots* also by cattle.

বকম *Bukum.* Shrub and climber. Moluccas, Ceylon, Coromandel, Bengal, (Serampore.) Flower largish, yellow, hot season; fruit cold season. Affords the *Red wood* of commerce, which is extensively exported as a dye wood.

বকুল *Bukul.* A tree. Moluccas, Ceylon. Both Peninsulas of India, Bengal, (Serampore,) Sylhet. Flower middle-sized, white, fragrant, hot season; fruit rainy season. A very ornamental tree, on account of its fragrant flowers generally found in our gardens.

বঙ্গ গন্ধিনা *Bunga-ghundeena.* A perennial. Cultivated about Calcutta. In Honorable Company's Garden flower rainy season. We use it as an article of diet, as leeks are used in Europe.

বচ *Buch.* মহব্বরী বচ *Muhubburee-buch.* A perennial. Moluccas, Cochin China. Both Peninsulas of India, Bengal, (Calcutta, Serampore.) Flower middle-sized, pale sulphur-coloured, rainy season; fruit December and November. In the Moluccas the young leaves and shoots are used as greens. (*Rumph.*) *Root* employed by us as a stimulant stomachic.

বজরা *Bujura.* An annual. Cultivated in India, especially over the higher lands on the Coast of Coromandel. Flower rainy season; fruit cold season. Cattle are fond of the straw, and the grain is a very essential article of food amongst the natives. (*Roxb.*)

বজুর *Bujoor.* A tree. Bengal. Flower March and April; fruit October and November.

বট *But.* *Banyan-tree,* radicant. Fruit-receptacles axillary, paired, sessile, as large as a middle-sized cherry, appearing and ripening hot season. Common all over India, in some places of an immense size. Lieut. Colonel Sykes mentions one at the village of Mhow, in the Poonah Collectorate, with 68 stems descending from the branches, and capable of affording shade, under a vertical sun, to 20,000 men. (*Madr. Journ. of Science, No.* 22.) *Bark* smooth, light ash-coloured. *Wood* light, white, and porous. *Leaves* used by the Brahmins to eat off, for which purpose they are joined together by inkles. *Birdlime* is prepared from the tenacious milky juice, which every part of the tree yields in abundance on being wounded. Birds eat the fruit, and the seeds grow the better for having passed through them. If they drop in the axils of the leaves of the Palmyra-tree, (Borasus flabelliformis, L.) they grow, and extend their descending parts so as an time to embrace entirely the Palmyra, except its upper parts, In very old ones the top thereof is just seen issuing from the trunk of the Banyan itself, as if it grew from thence, whereas it runs down through its centre, and has its roots in the ground, the Palm being the oldest. (*Roxb.*)

বড় কঙ্গি *Bura-kungi.* A perennial. Moluccas, Both Peninsulas of India, Bengal, Hindoosthan. Flower large, deep orange; cold season, fruit hot season.

বড় কট *Buro-kut.* A perennial. Coromandel, Concans, Bengal, (Serampore,) &c. Flower 3 lines long, white, rainy and cold season ; fruit cold season.

বড় কল্প *Buro-kulpa.* An annual. Ceylon, Deccan, Bengal, (Serampore.) New Holland. Flower middle-sized, pale blue, cold season ; fruit hot season.

বড় কান্থড় *Buro-kanoor.* A perennial. Moluccas. Both Concans, Lower Bengal. Common in gardens. Flower large, white, nearly inodorous, rainy and cold season ; fruit cold season. *Root* a good substitute for the Squill. (*O'Shaughnessy.*)

বড় কুকুর চিতা *Buro-kookoor-chita.* A tree. Peninsula of India, Bengal, (Serampore,) Uude Assam, Sylhet, Nepal. Flower small, yellowish-greenish, May and June ; fruit rainy season.

বড় কুন্দ *Buro-koondo.* A shrub. China, Cochin China, Courtallam, Monghyr, Hurdwar. Flower large, snow-white, very fragrant, March and April ; fruit none.

বড় কেরই *Buro-keruee.* An annual. Moluccas, Ceylon, Peninsula of India, Bengal, (Serampore.) Flower minute, greenish ; and fruit the whole year.

বড় কেশতি *Buro-keshuti.* An annual. Borders of the Circars, Bengal. Flower small, white, February and March ; fruit cold season.

বড় কেশুরিয়া *Buro-keshooreya.* A perennial. Bengal, (Serampore.) Flower and fruit rainy season.

বড় কোকসিম *Buro-kokesima.* An annual. Peninsula of India, Bengal, (Serampore,) Sylhet, China, Java. Flower small, yellowish, cold season; fruit February and March. The whole plant is strongly aromatic, somewhat smelling of turpentine, and is often used in cases of dyspepsia by us.

বড় গেঁদা *Buro-genda. African Marygold.* An annual. Mexico. Domesticated in India. Flower large, citron-coloured, cold season. Has a fetid smell.

বড় গোথুবি *Buro-gothoobee.* A perennial. Peninsula of India, Bengal, (Serampore,) Mauritius, China, Ascension. Flower and fruit rainy season.

বড় চনা *Buro-chuna.* Another name of ঝঞ্ঝনী আঁকরী *Jhunjhu-nee-ankuree.* See before.

বড় চালি *Buro-chali.* A tree. Peninsula of India, Mountains of Khassya, Monghyr and Morung, Bengal, (Serampore.) Flower small, greenish-white, throughout the year; fruit cold season.

বড় ছুঁচা *Buro-chhooncha.* A perennial. Peninsula of India, Bengal, (Serampore,) Nepal, Manilla, Macao. Flower and fruit rainy season.

বড় যবানী *Buro-yuvanee.* An annual. Bengal, (Serampore.) Flower and fruit rainy season.

বড় জালগাঁটী *Buro-jalgantee.* A perennial. Bengal, (Serampore,) &c. Flower rainy season; fruit cold season. Cattle are fond of it.

বড় ঝাঁঝি *Buro jhanjee.* An annual. Lower Egypt, Coromandel, Bombay, Bengal, (Serampore.) Flower smallish, yellow, and fruit rainy season.

বড় টগোর *Buro-tugur.* A shrub. Flower double, very fragrant during the night. More common in gardens.

বড় নীলপদ্ম *Buro-neel-pudma.* A perennial. Bengal, (Serampore.) Flower largish, blue, hot and rainy season; fruit rainy season.

বড়ন্দ *Burundo.* An annual. Bengal, (Serampore.) Flower rainy season; fruit cold season.

বড় পানচুলী *Buro-pan-choolee. Indian Buckbean.* An annual. Peninsula of India, Moluccas, Bengal, (Serampore,) &c.

Flower middle-sized, with a yellow tube, and a white-bearded limb, rainy and cold season; fruit cold season.

বড় পানী মরীচ *Buro-panee-murich.* An annual. Bengal, (Serampore.) Flower small, white, rainy season; fruit cold season.

বড় ফুটিকা *Buro-phootika.* A shrub. Moluccas, Sumatra, Cochin-China, Malay Islands. Both Peninsulas of India, Orissa, Jellasore, Khassya Mountains, Nepal. Flower large, red, and fruit whole year. *Berries* dye black.

বড় বহুয়ারি *Buro-buhooari.* A tree. Hindoosthan, Sylhet. Common throughout Guzerat. Flower small, white, cold season; fruit June and July. The fruit, while young and tender, is pickled, and is also eaten as a vegetable.

বড় বেত *Buro-bet.* Shrub and climber. Bengal, (Serampore,) &c. Flower rainy season; fruit cold season. The stems divested of the sheaths of the leaves are about as thick as a man's fore-finger, and employed for walking sticks.

বড় বেল *Buro-bel.* *Great double Arabian or Tuscan Jasmine.*

বড় মন্দা *Buro-munda.* Parasitic. A shrub. Peninsula of India, Bengal, (Serampore,) &c. Flower large, greenish orange-scarlet, and fruit nearly throughout the year.

বড় মসুর *Buro-musoor.* *Lentil Tare.* An annual. Europe. Cultivated in Bengal, and other adjoining provinces. Flower small, pale-blue, and fruit cold season.

বড় মাকাল *Buro-makal.* Shrub and climber. Both Peninsulas of India, Bengal, (Serampore,) Khassya Mountains, Deyra-Dhoon. Flower large, white, rainy season; fruit cold season. *Root* reckoned poisonous (*Roxb.*); with the *stem* much esteemed in diseases of cattle, as inflammation of the lungs, &c. (*Dr. Gibson.*)

বড় মেথি *Buro-methee.* An annual. S. France. Cultivated in India. Flower small, white, and fruit cold season. *Seeds* esteemed slightly tonic, and much eaten by the Indians.

বড় যোয়ান *Buro-joan.* An annual. Native place? Cultivated all over India. Flower small, white, cold season; fruit hot season. *Seeds* of an aromatic smell, a warm, pungent taste; much used by the Indians for medicinal and culinary purposes.

বড় রক্ত কম্বল *Buro-rukto-kumbul.* A perennial. Both Peninsulas of India, Bengal, (Serampore.) Flower large, intensely red, hot and rainy season, fruit rainy season.

বড় রাই *Buro-rai.* An annual. Bengal, (Serampore.) Cultivated on account of the oil of its seeds. Flower largish, yellow, December ; fruit February.

বড় রিঠা *Buro-ritha.* A tree. Peninsula of India, Bengal. Flower small, white, October and November ; fruit February and March. *Seeds* used medicinally, and for washing the finer kinds of silk.

বড় লুনিয়া *Buro-looniya. Common Purslane.* An annual. All over India, Ceylon, Java. &c. Flower small, yellow, rainy season ; fruit cold season.

বড় শন্ধি *Buro-sundhi.* A perennial. Bengal, (Serampore,) &c. Flower large, rose-coloured, or bluish white, hot and rainy season, fruit rainy season.

বড় সাদা মাখন শিম *Buro-sada-makhun-shim.* Perennial and climber. Pods about two feet long, often twenty-seeded. This variety is considered the most wholesome of them all, and is extensively used at the tables of Europeans, as well as by the Natives of Sylhet, where the plant is indigenous.

বড় শামা *Buro-shama.* An annual. Bengal, (Serampore,) &c. Flower rainy season ; fruit cold season.

বড় সালপানী *Buro-salpanee.* A shrub. Both Peninsulas of India, Bengal, (Soonderbuns, Calcutta, Serampore.) Assam. Flower smallish, pale rose, crimson-veined, rainy season ; fruit cold season.

বড় শালুক *Buro-shaluk.* A perennial. Africa. Both Peninsulas of India, Bengal, (Serampore,) &c. ; in short, like the other species, except N. rubra, found in every part of India, from 8° to 32° N. Lat. (*Royle.*) Flower large, white, of a vinous smell, rainy and cold season ; fruit hot season.

বড় শুঁঠী *Buro-shoonti.* An annual. Bengal, (Serampore,) Peninsula of India, New Holland, Cochin China. Flower rainy season.

বড় শোঙ্গ *Bursunga. Curry-leaf.* A small tree. Coromandel Assam, Kemaon. Flower small, white, fragrant, cold season ; fruit hot season. *Leaves* very fragrant, used for seasoning curries, stomachic, and tonic. Dried they retain these qualities, and are sold in the bazars. An infusion of them considered antemetic.

বড় শেলকাঁটা *Buro-shelkanta.* An annual. Mexico. Domesticated all over tropical India. Flower large, yellow, fruit January, February and March. *Seeds* narcotic, especially when smoked with tobacco. (*Gardener's, mag.* 6, *p.* 315;) In the W. Indies, they are used for many purposes, seemingly without much benefit. Lamp oil extracted from the seeds, employed by the poor in the Concans. (*Dr. Gibson.*)

বড় হল কশা *Buro-hulkusa.* An annual. Peninsula of India, Bengal, (Serampore,) Hindoosthan, Nepal. Flower small, white, rainy and cold season; fruit cold season.

বড় পিনি নটী *Buro-pini-nutee.* An annual, Peninsula of India, Bengal, (Serampore,) China. Flower rainy season; fruit cold season.

বন অচ *Bun-uch.* A small tree. Ataveesy-jungles, Bengal, (Serampore.) Flower small, white, hot and rainy season; fruit cold season.

বন আদা *Bun-ada.* A perennial. Coromandel, The Concans, Behar, Bengal. (Serampore,) Sylhet. Flower large, uniformly pale sulphur-coloured, July and August; fruit November and December. Has a strong camphoraceous smell, and yields the true *Cassumunar* of the shops, which is employed as a stimulant stomachic. (*Roxb.*)

There are three kinds of বন ওকড়া *Bun-okra.* viz :—

1. An undershrub. Flower middle-sized, rose-coloured, rainy season; fruit cold season. Both Peninsulas of India, Bengal, (Serampore,) Nepal.

2. An annual. Peninsula of India, Bengal, (Serampore.) Saharunpore. Flower small, yellow, rainy and cold season; fruit cold season.

3. An annual. Egypt. Most parts of India, (Serampore.) Flower small, white, February and March; fruit hot season.

বন কচু *Bun-kuchoo.* A perennial. Leaves uniformly green. Not cultivated. Seldom eaten by lower class of people.

বন কলমী *Bun-kulmee.* A perennial. China, Java, Ceylon,

Both Peninsulas of India, Bengal, (Serampore.) Flower largish, pale rose-coloured, with a dark purple eye, and fruit the whole year.

বন কলায় *Bun-kulay.* Undershrub and climber. Both, Peninsulas of India, Bengal. (Serampore,) Bolahat. Flower small, rose-coloured, rainy season; fruit cold season.

বন কাওয়া *Bun kaoa.* A shrub. Bengal, (Serampore,) Khassya Mountains, Assam, Nepal. Flower large, pure white, March, April and May; fruit hot season.

• বন কাপাস *Bun-kapas.* A biennial. Both Peninsulas of India, Bengal, (Serampore.) Flower large, sulphur, with a dark-purple eye, rainy and cold season; fruit cold season.

বন গমক *Bun-gumuk.* Annual and creeper. Coromandel, Bengal, (Serampore,) Saharunpore, Delhi, &c. Flower largish yellow, rainy and cold season; fruit cold season. On ripening it becomes aromatic.

বন গাব *Bun-gab.* A tree. Peninsula of India, Bengal, (Serampore, Monghyr.) Flower small, greenish-white, March and April; fruit rainy season.

বন গুয়া *Bun-gooa.* A tree. Chittagong. Flower minute, May to January; fruit April.

বন চাঁড়াল *Bun-charal.* An undershrub. Both Peninsulas of India, Bengal, (Serampore,) Assam, Kheree-jungle, Deyra-Dhoon, Kemaon. Flower small, dull-orange, rainy and cold season; fruit cold season.

বন চাঁদড় *Bun-chandur.* Shrub and climber. Tropical New Holland, Moluccas, Cochin China, Ceylon. Both Peninsulas of India, Bengal, (Serampore;) Sylhet. Flower small, white, rainy season; fruit cold season.

বন চালিতা *Bun-chalita.* A perennial. Sylhet, Burma, Lower Bengal, (Serampore.) Flower small, white, rainy season; fruit cold season.

বন চিচিঙ্গা *Bun-chichinga.* Annual and climber. Bengal, (Serampore.) Flower small, white, rainy and cold season; fruit cold season. Eaten by lower class of people.

বন যোয়ান *Bun-joan.* An annual. Lower Bengal, (Serampore.) Flower small, white, cold season; fruit hot season. *Seed* used as a medicine for cattle.

বন জাম *Bun-jam.* A shrub. Ceylon. Both Peninsulas of India; Bengal, (Serampore,) Nepal, Sumatra, Java. Flower smallish, pale rose-coloured, and fruit the whole year.

বন তেপরিয়া *Bun-tepuriya.* An annual. Tropical N. Holland, Moluccas, Cochin-China, Java, Ceylon, Peninsula of India, Bengal, (Serampore,) Hindoosthan, Nepal. Flower small, uniformly pale yellow, rainy and cold season; fruit cold season.

বন তুলসী *Bun-tulsee.* A biennial. Peninsula of India, Bengal, (Serampore.) Flower small, pale rose-coloured, rainy season; fruit cold season. Whole plant scentless.

বন নটি *Bun-nuti.* An annual. Peninsula of India, Bengal, (Serampore.) Flower minute, greenish, and fruit rainy season.

বন নারাঙ্গা *Bun-naranga.* A small tree. Circars, Bengal, (Serampore.) Flower small, yellow, fragrant, hot season; fruit rainy season.

বন নারাঙ্গী *Bun-narangee.* An annual. Moluccas. Both Peninsulas of India, Bengal, (Serampore.) Flower smallish, yellow, and fruit cold season.

বন নীল *Bun-neel.* A shrub. Mauritius, Bushire, Ceylon, Concan, Deccan, Deera, Coromandel, Kyouk Talong, Yenangheum, Segaen, Malloon, Tavoy, Bengal, (Serampore,) Monghyr, Delhi, Banks of the Jumna, Assam. Flower small, purple, rainy season; fruit cold season. *Roots* bitter, a decoction considered good in dyspepsia.

বন পটোল *Bun-putol.* Annual and climber. Both Peninsulas of India, Bengal, (Serampore.) Flower small, white, rainy season; fruit cold season. Unripe *fruit* very bitter, eaten by the poor.

বন পালঙ্গ *Bun-palung.* An annual. Coromandel, (Samulkota,) Bengal, (Serampore,) &c. Flower large, yellow, February and March; fruit hot season. Cattle are fond of every part of the plant, which on being wounded, discharges much milky juice that thickens into a substance like fresh, soft opium. (*Roxb.*)

বন পিড়িঙ্গ *Bun-piring.* An annual. Fields of Europe, Peninsula of India, Bengal, (Serampore,) Assam, Saharunpore. Flower small, white, and fruit cold season.

বন মল্লিকা *Bun-mullika. Single flowered Arabian Jasmine.* A twining plant.

22

বন মেথি *Bun-methee.* An annual. France, Italy, Greece, Bengal, (Serampore.) Flower minute, herewhite and fruit cold season.

বন যুঁই *Bun-jooen.* A shrub. New Holland, China, Moluccas. Both Peninsulas of India, Soonderbuns. Flower nearly 2 inches, pure white, with greenish-white tube, rainy and cold season.

বন বর্বটি *Bun-burbuti.* Perennial and twining plant. Coromandel, Common throughout the Concans, Bengal, (Serampore.) Flower large, deep rose-purple, cold season; fruit hot season. *Roots* tuberous, eaten by the poorer class.

বন রাই *Bun-rai.* An annual. Bengal, (Serampore.) Flower very small, yellow, and fruit the greater part of the year.

বন রাজ *Bun-raj.* A shrub. Mysore. Common on the ghauts and hilly parts of the Concans, Monghyr, Kheree Pass, Bengal, (Serampore.) Flower small, white, May and June; fruit cold season. *Bark* used for making matches. (*J. Grah.*)

বন লবঙ্গ *Bun-lubunga.* An annual. Both Peninsulas of India, Bengal, (Serampore.) Flower small, yellow, and fruit rainy season.

বন সিম *Bun-shim.* Perennial and twining plant. Common about Serampore. Flower smallish, purple. Seeds dark grey, mottled. Not cultivated.

বন সফেদ পুঁই *Bun sufed-pooin.* Perennial and twining plant. All over the jungles of India.

বন শুলফা *Bun-sulpha.* An annual. Europe, Neelgherries, Candesh, Bombay, Bengal, (Serampore, &c.) Nepal, Kemaon. Flower very small, pale rose-coloured, dark purple tipped, and fruit cold season.

বর্বটি *Burbuti.* Annual and twining plant. Commonly cultivated. Flower largish, rainy season; fruit cold season.

বসরাই গোলাব *Busurai-golab.* A shrub. S. Europe. Flower large, double rose, fragrant, February and hot season.

বরীথী *Burethee.* A perennial. Peninsula of India, Bengal, (Serampore,) Nepal. Flower and fruit rainy season.

বলা *Bula.* A small tree. Moluccas, Cochin-China, Soonderbuns. Flower hot and rainy season; fruit cold season.

বহুরা *Bahura.* A tree. Peninsula of India, Goalparrah, Sukanaghur, Goruckpur, Dhomtola, Morung Mountains. Flower small, greyish-green, offensively smelling, hot season; fruit cold season. *Wood* white, softish, durable. *Bark,* when wounded, gives out a large quantity of an insipid gum, resembling *Gum arabic.* Fruit (*Beleric myrobalans*) astringent tonic. *Kernels,* tasting like filberts, eaten by the natives and held to be intoxicating, when eaten in abundance. (*Roxb.*)

বহুয়ারি *Buhooari.* A small tree. Both Peninsulas of India, Bengal, Hindoosthan, Nepal, Egypt. Flower small, white, cold season; fruit May and June. Wood soft, and of little use except for fuel, and kindling fire by friction. Fruit eaten pickled or raw. Smell of the *nut,* when cut, heavy and disagreeable. Kernels tasting like fresh filberts. (*Roxb.*) The tree abounds in a transparent, glutinous juice.

বাঁশ *Bansh.* A tree. Mountains of India. Flower hot season. Much used in making huts &c. In Mysore and S. Concan the seeds are gathered for food by the poorer classes. (*Buch.*)

বাঁশ পাট নটি *Bansh-pata-nuti.* An annual. Bengal, (Serampore.) Flower minute, greenish, and fruit rainy season. The *leaves* and *tender tops* are eaten by the poorer classes in their curries.

বাঁশিনি বাঁশ *Bashini-bansh.* A tree. Has a larger cavity, and is used chiefly for making baskets.

বাকস *Bukus.* A shrub. Java, Ceylon. Both Peninsulas of India, Bengal, (Serampore,) Sylhet, Nepal, &c. Flower 14 lines, white, tinged with sulphur at the throat, and at the limb with dark purple lines and spots, cold season; fruit February. *Wood* soft, considered very fit for making charcoal for gunpowder. (*Roxb.*) *Flowers, leaves.* and *roots* bitterish, subaromatic, and considered antispasmodic.

বাকসা *Buksa.* An annual. Bengal, (Serampore.) Flower rainy season; fruit cold season. Cattle are fond of this grass.

বাকাজ্জ'ন *Bukarjun.* Hind, *Bukayun.* A tree. Persia, Nepal, Kemaon. Cultivated in our gardens. Flower smallish, lilac, fragrant, and fruit the whole year.

বাঘ অঙ্কড়া *Bagh-ankra.* A tree. Coromandel, Cochin, Bombay, Guzerat, Malay Peninsula, Cochin China, Assam, Khassya Mountains, &c., up to the base of the Himalaya. Flower middle-sized, whitish-yellowish, fragrant, hot season; fruit rainy season. *Wood* beautiful. *Fruit* edible, somewhat astringent.

বাঘ আচড়া *Bagh-achura.* Shrub and climber. Peninsula of India, Bengal, (Serampore.) Flower small, greenish-white, March and April; fruit cold season. Makes impenetrable hedges.

বাঘ লতা *Bagha-luta.* Same as তিলিয়া করা *Tiliyakura.*

বাঘ নখো শিম *Bagh-nukho-shim.* Flower white, largish.

বাঘ নলা *Bagh-nula.* An annual. Java, Ceylon, Peninsula of India, Bengal, (Serampore.) Flower largish, deep-blue, rainy season; fruit cold season.

বাঘ ভেরাণ্ডা *Bagh-bharanda.* A shrub. Cuba, S. America, Domesticated in India. Flower small, green, and fruit the whole year. *Seeds* purgative and occasionally emetic. An expressed *oil* is obtained from them, which is reckoned a valuable external application in itch and herpes; it is also used a little diluted, in chronic rheumatism. The varnish used by the Chinese for covering boxes is made by boiling this oil with oxide of iron. The *leaves* are considered rubefacient and discutient. The *milky-juice* is supposed to be detergent and healing, and dyes linen black. (*Ainslie.*)

বাঙ্গড়া *Bangra.* Same as কেশ রাজ *Kesho-raj.*

বঙ্গ এলাচ *Bunga-elacha.* A perennial. Khassya Mountains. Flower large, yellow, March and April; fruit rainy season.

বাড়্যালা *Baryala.* A shrub. Both Peninsulas of India, Bengal, (Serampore.) Flower middle-sized, yellow, rainy and cold season; fruit cold season. The *mucilage* of this plant, mixed with rice, is used to alleviate dysentery.

বাতাবি নেবু *Batavi-neboo.* *Shaddock, Pumplemuss.* A small tree. Moluccas, Sunda Islands. Cultivated in India. Flower large, white, fragrant, February and March; fruit September, October and November.

বাদাম *Badam.* *Country Almond tree.* Moluccas. Both Peninsulas of India, Bengal, (Serampore.) Flower small, purplish-green, hot season; fruit rainy season. *Wood* good. Kernels palatable.

বানর কলায় *Banur-kulay.* Biennial and twining plant. Madagascar, Bourbon, Mauritius, Ceylon, Peninsula of India,

Bengal, (Serampore,) Khassya and Monghyr Hills, Assam, Mussoorie, Nepal. Flower small, yellow, rainy and cold season; fruit cold season. Eaten by cattle.

বানর লাঠি গাছ *Banur-lati-gachh.* সোনালু *Sonaloo.* A tree, Moluccas. Both Peninsulas of India, Bengal, (Serampore,) Assam, Oudh. Foot of the Himalayas. Flower large, bright yellow fragrant, May and June; fruit (বানর লাঠি *Banur-lati,*) February and March. The sweetish secretion surrounding the seeds is slightly aperient.

বাবলা *Babula.* A tree. Peninsula of India, Bengal, (Serampore,) Sukanaghur, Saharunpore. Flower small, bright-yellow, fragrant, May and October; fruit March. Produces, with A. speciosa, and Vachellia Farnesiana, a gum, which is used as a substitute for Gum Senegal, and Gum Arabic. *Wood* strong, tough, durable, making excellent knees and crooked timber in ship-building. *Bark* astringent, used for tanning leather, and to dye various shades of brown. A decoction of the bark employed as a substitute for soap. (*Roxb.*) *Seeds* and *pods* of great value to the shepherd in the hot season, as food for his flock, when grass is scarce. (*Dr. Gibson.*) This officer suggested some years ago to plant the waste part of the Deccan with this tree, as it grows rapidly and requires no water.

বাবুই তুলসী *Babooi-toolsee.* An undershrub. Peninsula of India, Bengal, (Serampore,) Hindoosthan, Oudh, &c. Flower small, white, and fruit nearly the whole year. Whole plant aromatic, fragrant. The *seeds* steeped in water swell into a pleasant jelly, which is used by us in cases of catarrh, dysentery, chronic diarrhœa, &c. and is very nourishing and demulcent.

বামন হাটি *Bamun-hatee.* A shrub. Prome, Ava, Tavoy, Peninsula of India, Bengal, (Serampore,) Sylhet, &c. Flower more than four inches long, greenish-white, April, May and from August to January; fruit January and February.

বালকু বাঁশ *Balkoo-bansh.* The same as পলু বাঁশ *Puloo-bansh.*

বাসন্তী *Basuntee.* মাধবি *Madhubee.* মাধবি লতা *Madhubee-lata.* Shrub and climber. Coromandel, The Ghauts, Prome, Martaban, Bengal, (Serampore,) Goalpara, Hindoosthan, Nepal. Flower middle-sized, sweet-scented, white, with a tinge of sulphur, rainy and cold season; fruit cold season.

বিচ তাড়কা *Bich-taruka.* Shrub and twining plant. Coromandel, Malabar-hill, Malabar, Deccan, Bengal, (Serampore,)

Hindoosthan, Deyra Dhoon, Java, Isle of France. Flower large deep rose-coloured, rainy and cold season; fruit March. The upper side of the leaves is used to act as a discutient; the under, or white side, as a maturant.

বিছুটী *Bichhutee.* Shrub and climber. Ceylon, Peninsula of India, Bengal, (Serampore.) Flower small, greenish, and fruit the whole year. The *hair* of this plant stings like that of the common nettle. The *root* is used in preparing medicine.

বিনা *Bina.* Between the tropics all over the world. N. Holland, Penang, Singapore, Moluccas, Soonderbuns, &c. Flower small, dingy-yellow, hot season; fruit none. The *bark* is in general use in *Rio Janeiro* for tanning. *(Lindl.*

বিল ঝঝুন *Bil-jhunjhun.* An annual. Moluccas, Peninsula of India. Taong-Dong, Bengal, (Serampore,) Assam, Kheree jungle, Deyra-Dhoon. Flower large, bright yellow, cold season; fruit hot season. Fibres of the bark employed in many places in the manufacture of cordage and canvas.

বিল নালিতা *Bil-nalita.* See জঙ্গলি পাট *Junglee-pat.*

বিল পাট *Bil-pat.* See টিকিও পড়া *Tikee-opra.*

বিল রাই *Bil-rai.* An annual. Bengal, (Serampore.) Flower very small, yellow, rainy season; fruit cold season.

বিল লতা *Bil-luta.* A shrub. Bengal, (Serampore,) Hindoosthan, Deyra-Dhoon, Kheree Pass. Kemaon. Flower small, tinged with deep rose, cold season; fruit hot season. The plant posses-ses a strong, heavy, aromatic smell, and a bitterish taste.

বিলাতি আনান্নাস *Bilati-anannas.* A perennial. Moluccas? S. China? Flower in May and June, when from 10 to 15 years old, and then from 20 to 30 feet high (*Roxb.*)

বিলাতি আমড়া *Bilati-amra. Otaheyti Apple-tree.* Society Islands. Cultivated in India. Flower small, greenish-yellow, March; fruit December and January. *Fruit* eaten by all nation.

বিলাতি আলু *Bilati-aloo. Potatoe.* A perennial. West Coast of S. America. Cultivated all over the world. Flower middle-sized, white or blue, and fruit cold season.

বিলাতি পির্তসিল্লি *Bilati-pitursilli.* A biennial. Sardinia, Greece, Turkey, near constantinople, &c. Flower small, yellow-ish, cold season; fruit hot season. Cultivated in India.

বিলাতি মেন্দি *Bilati-mendee.* A shrub. S. Europe, Common in gardens. Flower smallish, white, fragrant, hot season; fruit none. Used as a hedge-plant in Egypt. (*Macullough.*) *Berries* eaten in Syria.

বিলিম্বি *Bilimbi.* A small tree. Moluccas. Cultivated. Flower small, reddish-brown, hot season; fruit rainy season. Fruit pickled, or preserved with sugar.

বিষ *Bish* is a most virulent poison, used in the northern part of Hindoosthan for destroying tigers by means of poisoned arrows, shot from bows fixed near the tracks leading to their watering places.

বিষ বাঁশ *Bish-bansh.* A tree. Peninsula of India, Chittagong Mountains. Flower rainy season; fruit cold season.

বিষমান *Biskman.* A perennial. Bengal, (Serampore.) Flower rainy season.

বুঁইচ *Booinck.* A shrub. Peninsula of India, Bengal, (Serampore,) Hindoosthan and northwards to Deyra-Dhoon. Flower minute, greenish, cold season; fruit hot season. Fruit eaten by us.

বুট কলায় *Boot-kalay.* The same as চনা *Chuna.*

বুড়ি গোপানা *Boori-gopana.* A perennial. Tanjore. The Concans, Bengal, (Serampore.) Flower large, pale blue, expanding in the evening, drooping the next morning, nearly the whole year; fruit cold season.

বেগ পুরা *Beg-poora.* *Common Citron.* A small tree. Foot of the Himalaya, Garrow-Hills, &c. Cultivated. Flower white, tinged with red, fragrant, hot season; fruit rainy season.

বেগুন *Begoon Brinjal. Egg-plant.* A perennial. All over India. Flower largish, violet, cold season; fruit hot season. Eaten by all nation.

বেত *Bet.* Shrub and climber Bengal, (Serampore,) Coromandel, S. Concan, Ram Ghaut, &c. Flower rainy season; fruit cold season. Yields the common ratans.

বেত রঙ্গ *Bet-rung.* An undershrub. Bengal, (Calcutta, Serampore.) Taong-Dong. Flower 16 lines, deep rose-coloured, with a white tube, and a purple throat, rainy and cold season; fruit cold season.

বেতু শাক *Bettoo-shak.* An annual. Entirely green.

বেনা যোনি *Bena-yoni.* An annual. Bengal, (Serampore,) &c. Flower rainy season; fruit cold season.

বেলা *Bela.* *Double-flowered Arabian Jasmine. A twining plant.*

বেল *Bel.* A tree. Coromandel, Malabar Hill, Bombay, Elephanta, Bengal, (Serampore,) Assam, Common about the Pagodas, as the Hindus have a deep reverence for this tree. Flower middle-sized, greenish-white, fragrant, May; fruit October and November. The *fruit* is nutritious, warm, cathartic, delicious, exquisitely fragrant. Its aperient and detersive qualities, and its efficacy in removing habitual costiveness, have been proved by constant experience. The *bark of the root* is sometimes used by the Hindus in compound decoctions against intermittent fevers; while the fresh expressed *juice of the leaves*, diluted, is praised in catarrhs and feverishness—the *leaves* in a poultice against ophthalmias and a *decoction of the immature dried fruit* against diarrhœa, and dysentery. The *mature fruit*, mixed with tamarind juice, forms a sort of antifebrile sherbet. The astringent *rind of the fruit* is used in dyeing yellow, while the glutinous and tenacious matter which surrounds the seeds is considered an excellent addition to mortar, especially in well-building.

বেহড় বাঁশ *Behoor-bansh.* A tree. Bengal, (Calcutta, Serampore,) &c. Flower June. Grows to a pretty large size, has a smaller cavity than any of the other bamboos, is strong, and consequently adapted for various purposes.

বেহুয়া *Behooa.* An annual. Peninsula of India, Ceylon, Bengal, (Serampore,) New Holland, Mauritius, Egypt, Greece, Lombardy, Manilla, China. Flower and fruit rainy season.

ব্যাকুড় *Byakoor.* A shrub. All over India. Flower middle-sized, blue, and fruit the whole year.

ভাঙ্গড়া *Bhangra.* An undershrub. Both Peninsulas of India, Bengal, (Serampore,) Sutanaghur. Flower small, dark purple; and fruit nearly whole year.

ভাঁট *Bhant.* A shrub, Both Peninsulas of India, Bengal, (Serampore,) Oudh, &c. Flower large, white, tinged with rose on the inside, February and March; fruit April and May.

ভাট শোলা *Bhat-sola.* An annual. Bengal, (Serampore.) Flower middle-sized, bright yellow, rainy season; fruit cold season.

ভুঁই কামড়ি *Bhooin-kamri.* A perennial. Peninsula of India, Umerapura, Bengal, (Serampore.) Flower small, bright yellow, and fruit cold season.

There are two kinds of ভুঁই কুমড়া *Bhooin-koomra.*

1. Perennial and climber. Banks of the Megna, where the inhabitants use the *root* as a substitute for Calumba-root. It has been sent to England as the real Calumba of Mozambique. Flower large, white. In Honorable Company's Garden flower rainy season. (*Roxb.*)

2. Shrub and twining plant. New Holland. Java, Guinea, Cayenne, Banks of the Orinoco, Both Peninsulas of India, Bengal, (Serampore.) Sylhet, Assam. Flower large, rose-coloured, with a dark purple eye, cold season; fruit hot season. *Root* cathartic. Cattle eat it.

ভুঁই ওকড়া *Bhooin-okra.* See ছোট ওকড়া *Chhoto-okra.*

ভুঁই চাঁপা *Bhooin-champa.* A perennial. Native place uncertain. Commonly cultivated in gardens on account of the beauty and fragrance of its large purplish-white flowers, which appear in March and April; fruit none. *Roots* warmly aromatic.

ভুঁই জাম *Bhooin-jam.* A perennial. Interior of Bengal. Flower small, pale-whitish-yellow. February and March.

ভুঁই ডালিম *Bhooin-dalim.* A perennial. Interior of Bengal. Flower large, reddish greenish-white, February and March: fruit June and July.

ভুঁই ডুমুর *Bhooin-doomoor.* A shrub. Creeping. Bengal, (Serampore.) Fruit—receptacles axillary, solitary, peduncled, obovate, roughish, the size of the point of the little finger, appearing and ripening the whole year.

ভুঁই পাট *Bhooin-pat.* An annual. New Caledonia, Moluccas, Timor, Java, Ceylon. Both Peninsulas of India, Bengal, (Serampore,) &c. Flower small, white, and fruit February, March and April.

ভূত ভৈরবী *Bhoot-bhairabee.* A shrub. Bengal, (Serampore,) Goalpara, Morung, Nepal, Kemaon. Flower minute, greenish-white, rainy season; fruit cold season. The whole plant has a heavy, unpleasant smell, nearly the same as some of the other species of this genus.

ভু তুলসী *Bhoo-tulsee.* See কোক বরাদী *Koka-baradee.*

ভুট *Bhoot.* মক্কা *Mukka. Maize. Indian Corn.* An annual. Tropical America. Cultivated all over India, &c. Flower rainy and cold season; fruit cold season.

ভুমি নিম *Bhoomi-nim.* An annual. Peninsula of India, Bengal, (Serampore.) Flower smallish, pink-coloured, rainy season; fruit cold season.

ভুট রাজ *Bhoot-raj.* Perennial and climber. Bengal, (Serampore,) Peninsula of India. Flower rainy season.

ভেরাণ্ডা *Bherunda. Palma Christi. Castor-oil plant.* A shrub. Greece, N. Africa, India. Much cultivated. *Seeds* used by dyers to mix with colours and render them permanent. The oil often used in lamps. *Leaves* a favourite food of some silk worms.

ভেলা *Bhela.* A tree. Coromandel. Common throughout the Concans, and in Goozerat, (whence, a considerable quantity of nuts is exported.) Berar, Sylhet, Assam, extending to Deyra-Dhoon and Kyarda. Flower small, green, May, June and July; fruit January and February. The *wood* of the *Marking-nut Tree* is of no use, partly on account of its softness, and partly because its abundance of acrid juice renders it dangerous to work. *Bark* mildly astringent, giving out in decoction a deep colour, which dyes brown of various shades. Wounded, it yields a dirty looking, brownish, soft gum, slowly dissolving in the mouth without much taste. The *receptacle* of the fruit roasted in ashes, is eaten by the poorer class, and tastes like roasted apples, whereas raw, it is astringent and acrid, leaving a painful sensation for some time on the tongue. The *green nuts*, well-pounded into a paste, make good bird-lime. The pure black, *acrid juice* of the nuts is employed to remove rheumatic pains, aches and sprains, though in tender constitutions it often produces inflammation, doing much more harm than good; but in general the rubbing on of the oil has not this effect, and is then an efficacious remedy. It is generally employed to mark all sorts of cotton-cloth. By a mixture of quick lime and water, the colour is improved, prevented from running, and fixed.

ভোরা *Bhora.* A tree. Mauritius, Madagascar, Ceylon,

Java, Arabia Felix, Malabar, Soonderbuns, &c. Flower largish, white, sweet-scented. In Honorable Company's Garden flower April and May; fruit cold season. *Wood* dark reddish, hard and durable.

মক্কা *Mukka.* See ভুট *Bhoot.*

মটর *Mutur. Pea.* An annual. Native place unknown. Cultivated in India. Flower large, white, or variegated with red, and fruit cold season.

মথরা *Muthura.* A shrub. Bengal, (Serampore.) Flower small, purple, hot and rainy season; fruit cold season.

মদন নির্ব্বিষি *Mudun-nirbishi.* Hind. *Kanjonboora.* A perennial. Bengal. Flower large, white, faintly purple tinged towards the apex, with the lip lilac, and at the middle dark-purple, June and July; fruit none. *Root* used as a medicine for cattle.

মন *Muna.* A shrub. Coromandel, S. Concan, Ceylon, Bengal, (Serampore.) Flower large, bright-yellow, and fruit nearly the whole year.

ময়চা *Moicha.* A small tree. Sylhet, Lower Bengal, (Serampore.) Flower small, greenish-white, March; fruit rainy season.

ময়না *Moyna.* A shrub. Bengal, (Serampore.) Flower small, pale greenish, March and April; fruit rainy season. Fruit eaten.

মসিনা *Musina.* An annual. Europe. Flower smallish, sky-blue; cold season; fruit hot season. Much cultivated in N. India for the seeds, from which the oil is extracted.

মহব্বরি বচ *Muhubburee-buch.* See বচ *Buch.*

মহা তিতা *Maha-tita.* See কাল মেঘ *Kalo-megh.*

মহুয়া *Muhooa.* A tree. Mountainous parts of the Circars, Bengal, Malabar Hill, Bombay. Throughout the Concans, Guzerat, Malwa. Flower middle-sized, white, with a tinge of green and cream-colour, March and April; fruit July and August. *Wood* hard, very strong, and proper for naves of wheel-carriages. *Flowers* eaten raw by the poorer people. An ardent spirit is distilled from them. The *seeds* yield by expression a large quantity of concrete oil, which is used to adulterate ghee, for frying cakes, and by the poorer people to burn. There is frequently to be found a drop of whitish, soft, tasteless resin on the apices of the flowers, before they open.

There are two kinds of মাকড়জালী *Makur-jalee.*

1. An annual, Bengal, (Serampore,) &c. Flower rainy season; fruit cold season. Cattle are very fond of this grass.

2. An annual. Tropical America, Africa, Moluccas. Both Peninsulas of India, Bengal, (Serampore.) Flower and fruit nearly throughout the year. Cattle are fond of this grass.

মাখন শিম *Makhun-shim.* Perennial and climber. Flower large, rainy season; fruit cold season. Its half-grown pods afford a passable vegetable.

মাখাল *Makhal. Colocynth-plant.* An annual. Peninsula of India, Banks of the Jumna, Kemaon, Japan. Flower yellow, rainy season; fruit cold season.

মাদুর কাটি *Madoor-katee.* A perennial. Peninsula of India, Bengal, (Serampore.) Flower and fruit rainy season. Those elegant, useful, durable, large mats so common on the floors of rooms in and about Calcutta, are made of the culm of this plant. When green, they are split into three or four pieces, which on drying contract so much as to bring the margins in contact, or to overlop each other. In this state they are wove.

মাধবী *Madhubee.* মাধবী লতা *Madhubee-lata.* See বাসন্তী *Basuntee.*

মান কচু *Man-kuchoo.* A perennial. Various parts of India. In Bengal it is cultivated for its esculent stems and small pendulous tubers, these being very generally eaten by people of all ranks in curries, &c. Flower September, October and November.

মান গিরি *Man-giri.* Petioles darker-coloured. This as well as a seldom produce ripe seeds.

মারুয়া *Murooa.* An annual. Cultivated. Flower rainy season; fruit cold season.

মারহাটা তিগা *Marhata-tiga.* An annual. Moluccas, Peninsula of India, Bengal, (Serampore.) Flower small, yellow, rainy and cold season, fruit cold season.

মাল আঁকড়া *Mal-ankura.* An annual. Ceylon, Peninsula of India, Bengal, (Serampore,) &c. Egypt, W. Indies. Flower and fruit nearly throughout the year.

মালা *Mala.* Perennial and climber. Peninsula of India,

Goalpara, Bengal, (Serampore,) Deyra-Dhoon, Cashmere. Flower small, yellowish-green; and fruit throughout the year.

মালাকা আমরুল *Malaka-amrool,* A tree. Moluccas. Cultivated. Flower large crimson, hot season; fruit rainy season.

মালাকা ঝাঁঝি *Malaka-jhanji.* An annual. Standing water in S. Europe and Bengal. Flower small, white. Has been introduced into Honorable Company's Garden.

মাষ কলায় *Mash-kalay.* An annual. Circars, Travancore, Malabar, Bengal, (Serampore,) in a cultivated state only. Flower middle sized, yellow, and fruit cold season. This species is the most esteemed of all the liguminous plants, and bears the highest price. Eaten by us. Its produce is about thirty-fold. Cattle eat the straw.

মাষানী *Mashanee.* Perennial and climber. Bengal, (Serampore.) Flower minute, deep reddish violet, rainy season; fruit cold season.

মিঠা কামরাঙ্গা *Mita-kumrunga.* A tree. Ripe fruit sweet. Eaten by us.

মিঠা নেবু *Mita-neboo.* Cultivated.

মুক্ত জুড়ি *Mookto-joori.* An annual. Peninsula of India, Bengal, (Serampore,) &c. Flower small, greenish, rainy season; fruit cold season. *Root,* bruised in hot water, cathartic. A decoction of the *leaves* laxative. Cats are as much affected by the roots as by those of Valerian. (*Nimmo.*)

মুক্ত পাতী *Mookto-patee.* See পাতী পাতী *Patee-Patee.*

মুগানী *Mooganee.* A perennial. Coromandel, Common in the Deccan and Bengal, (Serampore.) Flower small, yellow, and fruit cold season. Cultivated. Seeds gathered and eaten by the poor. Affords good fodder.

মুঙ্গ ফল্লী *Moong-phullee.* See আটকে কলায় *Atke-kulay.*

মুঠ *Moot.* An annual. Coromandel, Oudh. Cultivated in the Deccan, Goozerat and the Upper Provinces as fodder. Flower small, yellow, and fruit cold season.

মুড় মুড়ী *Moor-moori.* An annual. Bengal, (Serampore,) Peninsula of India. Flower and fruit rainy season.

মুথ *Mootho.* A perennial. Arabia, Ceylon, Peninsula of India, Bengal, (Serampore,) Kemaon, Java, China, Manilla, New

Holland. Flower and fruit rainy season. *Roots* tuberous, sold in the bazars, and used by perfumers on account of their fragrance. Cattle eat the grass. Hogs are remarkably fond of the root. In medicine it is used as a tonic and stimulant, and has been employed in the treatment of cholera.

মুন্দী *Mundee.* An annual. Peninsula of India, Bengal, (Serampore,) Hindoosthan, Kemaon. Flower small, purplish, cold season; fruit March. Whole plant very fragrant.

মূর্ব্বা *Moorba. Bowstring Hemp.* A perennial. Peninsula of India, Bengal, (Serampore,) &c. Flower middle-sized, greenish-white, somewhat fragrant, and fruit rainy season. This plant yields fibres of a fine and very strong quality, fitted for bowstrings, fishing lines, as well as for cordage, which, indeed, is made from it on the Coromandel coast. The fine fibres, called China grass, are made from this plant, which is a profitable cultivation in sandy soils of S. India.

মূলা *Moola. Common garden-radish.* Annual and biennial, China, Japan, W. Asia. Flower purplish-white, February and March; fruit April. Eaten by all nation.

মেন্দি *Mendi.* A small tree. Moluccas, Peninsula of India, Bengal, (Serampore,) Hindoosthan, &c. Exists in a cultivated state in N. Africa and most parts of the Oriental region. Flower small, pale greenish, fragrant; and fruit the whole year. This is the *Henna-plant* of Egypt. The fresh *leaves,* beaten up with Catechu, dye the nails and skin of a reddish orange colour, which is much admired by the women of India and Egypt. The fresh made paste is laid on at bed-time, and removed in the morning, when the colour remains till the nails or epidermis are renewed or removed. The leaves are also used for dyeing skins and maroquins reddish yellow, and for many other purposes. They contain no tannin.

মেরাড়ু *Meradoo.* See গারুড়ু *Garoodoo.*

মেলেঞ্চা *Melencha.* An annual. Bengal, Peninsula of India. Flower and fruit cold season.

মেষ্টা *Mesta.* The *Roselle* plant, or *Red Sorrel* of the W. Indies. An annual. W. Indies. Cultivated in India. Flower large, pale, sulphur, with a dark brown eye, rainy season; fruit cold season. From the fleshy, acid, red calyxes are prepared excellent jellies and tart fruits.

মেষ্টা পাট *Mesta-pata.* Flower large, sulphur, with a dark-brown eye, rainy season; fruit cold season. *Leaves* acidulous, eaten by the poor. Fibres of the *bark* used for cordage.

মৈনা *Myna.* See কোদ *Koda.*

মনসা সিজ *Munsa-sij.* A small tree. Moluccas, Peninsula of India, Bengal, (Serampore.) Flower middle-sized, greenish-yellow, rainy season. *Root,* mixed up with black-pepper, used against snake bites.

মোম চীনা *Mom-cheena.* See চেলাট পিপ্পল *Chelat-pipul.*

মোরঙ্গ এলাচী *Morung-elachee.* A perennial. Morung Mountains. Flower middle-sized, pale yellow, the lip tinged with red down the middle, hot season; fruit September. *Seeds* spicy, used for medicinal, and other purposes.

মৌ আলু *Mou-aloo.* Perennial and twining plant. Bengal, (Serampore,) Goa, &c. Flower small, whitish, rainy season. Roots about two pounds or more in weight, not cultivated, but dug up in the woods during the cold season, and carried for sale to the bazars.

রক্ত করবী *Rukto-kurubee.* A small tree. Flower single, deep-red.

রক্ত কাঞ্চন *Rukto-kanchun.* A tree. Bengal, (Serampore,) Pateram, Monihari, Puraniya. Four petals light purple; the fifth deep purple, tinged with cream and red. Flower large, February and March; fruit rainy season.

রক্ত কামলতা *Rukto-kamaluta.* Annual and twining plant. North and South America, Mauritius, E. Indies, northwards as far as Deyra-Dhoon. Flower deep red.

রক্ত গরানিয়া আলু *Rukto-guraniya-aloo.* Perennial and twining plant. Flower small, whitish, rainy season. Holds the third rank among the yams.

There are two kinds of রক্ত চন্দন *Rukto-chundun.*

1. A tree. Coromandel, Paulghaut Mountains. In Honorable Company's Garden flower hot season. From this tree is obtained the *red Sandal-wood,* chiefly employed by dyers and colour-manufacturers.

2. A tree. Moluccas. Both Peninsulas of India, Bengal, (Serampore,) Sylhet, Assam. Flower small, yellow, fragrant,

hot season; fruit rainy and cold season. Inner *wood* of large trees deep red, hard, durable and yielding a dye, with which the Hindus; after religious bathing, mark their foreheads. *Seeds* bright scarlet, and on account of their equality (each of them weighing four grains) used by goldsmiths and jewellers for weights.

রক্ত চিতা *Rukto-chita.* A shrub. Moluccas. Both Peninsulas of India, Common in gardens. Flower middle-sized, bright red, rainy and cold season; fruit hot season.

রক্ত পদ্ম *Rukto-pudmo.* Flower rose-coloured.

রক্ত পিট *Rukto-pit.* Shrub and climber. Moluccas, Both Peninsulas of India, Hills of Bengal, Assam, Nepal, Kemaon. Flower small, greenish, offensively smelling, cold season; fruit hot season. *Bark* used for cordage. According to Rumphius, the Amboyna fishermen use the long climbing stems instead of ropes.

রক্ত পুঁই *Rukto-pooin.* Perennial and twining plant. Flower small, red, January, February, and March; fruit hot season.

রক্ত বন পুঁই *Rukto-bun-pooin*, when wild.

রক্ত শিম *Rukto-shim.* Stem and the large flowers purple. Pods deep purple.

রক্ত শিমুল *Rukto-shimool. Red Cotton Tree.* Extends from one end of India to the other, particularly along the foot of the Himalayas. Flower very large, deep red, February and March; fruit April and May. *Bark* of the root used in Java as an emetic. (*Blume.*) *Wood* light, white, spongy, frequently used in India for floating rafters. (*Royle.*)

রক্ত সেলেঞ্চি *Rukto-shelenchi.* An annual. Bengal, (Serampore.) Flower minute, crimson, rainy and cold season; fruit cold season.

রঙ্গণ *Rungun.* A shrub. Hindoosthan, Common in Salsette. On the poor uncultivated land between Indapoor and Dasgaum, S. Concan. ((*J. Grah.*) Flower large, bright scarlet, the whole year; fruit cold season.

রঙ্গপুর নেবু *Rungpore-neboo.* Round, smooth-skinned Lime. Cultivated.

রঙ্গ মাখন শিম *Runga-makhun-shim.* Perennial and climber. Cultivated.

রজনী গন্ধা *Rujuni-gundha.* **A perennial. No doubt a native of Mexico or S. America. Gardens in India, Ceylon and Java. Flower large, white, fragrant, rainy season; fruit none.**

রসন ঝাঁঝি *Ruson-jhanji.* **An annual. Coromandel, The Concans, Bengal, (Serampore,) Sylhet. Flower very small, rainy season; fruit cold season.**

রশুন *Rushoon. Common Garlic.* **A perennial. Sicily. Cultivated in gardens. Flower small, white, hot season.**

রাঁধুনী *Radhunee.* An annual. Cultivated all over Bengal, at Singapore, Prome, &c. Native place? Flower small, white, February; fruit March and April. *Seeds* used for culinary and medicinal purposes. The *leaves,* though of an unpleasant smell, are now and then used as a substitute for Parsley by Europeans.

রাখাল ফুল *Rakhal-phul.* A shrub. Peninsula of India, Bengal, (Serampore.) Flower small, white, rainy season; fruit cold season. *Root* used by the Telinga physicians in substance to stop diarrhœas. Fruit eaten.

রাখাল শশা *Rakhal-Susha.* Perennial and climber. Both Peninsulas of India, Bengal, (Serampore,) Khassya Mountains, Sirmore. Flower small yellowish, rainy and cold season; fruit cold season; The ripe and unripe *fruit,* as well as the boiled *roots* eaten.

রাঙ্গা শাক *Ranga-shak.* লাল শাক *Lal-shak.* An annual. Bengal, (Serampore,) Assam, &c. Flower small, greenish or reddish, and fruit rainy season. Varieties of this species many, tolerably permanent, differing chiefly in colour from green with the slightest tinge of red, to rufous, liver coloured, and bright red.

রাম কলা *Ram-kula. Wild plantain.* Flower large, yellowish-whitish, and fruit throughout the year. A native of the E. Indies, cultivated every where within the Tropics.

রাম গুয়া *Ram-gooa.* A tree. S. Concan, Chittagong, Sylhet. In Honorable Company's Garden flower February and March; fruit rainy season.

রাম তরাই *Ramturay.* See ঢেঁড়স *Dhenroos.*

রাম তিল *Ram-til.* An annual. Abyssinia, Mysore, Deccan, where it is commonly cultivated for the sake of the oil it affords.

Lower Bengal. Flower large, bright-yellow, cold season; fruit February and March.

রাম তুলসী *Ram-tulsee.* A shrub. Only found in gardens. Diffuses a very strong degree of fragrance. Flower white, pale-yellow, and fruit nearly the whole year.

রাম বেগুণ *Ram-begoon.* A perennial. Cochin China, Penang, Singapore, Coromandel, S. Concan, Bengal, (Serampore.) Flower largish, white, rainy season; fruit cold season.

রাম হোগলা *Ram-hogla.* A perennial. Peninsula of India, Bengal, (Serampore.) N. India. Flower rainy season. *Leaves* used for making mats.

রিঠা *Ritha.* A tree. Bengal. Flower small, white, February and March; fruit cold season. *Fruit* used for washing.

রীঠা *Reeta.* Shrub and Climber. Peninsula of India, Banks of the Attran, Moulmein, Bengal, (Serampore,) Sylhet, Assam, Nepal. Flower small, white, rainy season; fruit cold season. The thick, succulent *legumes* are sold in the bazar, and used as soap for washing the hair, &c. They are also employed by Hindus for marking the forehead &c. The *leaves* are acid, and used in cookery instead of tamarinds.

রুমী মস্তকী *Roomee-mastuki.* See কুন্দ রুমী *Koondoo-roomee.*

রোহণ *Rohuna. Red-Wood tree.* A tree. Central and Southern Provinces of India. In considerable abundance in various parts of Guzerat; also at the Sindwah Ghat, and in the Adjunta and Jowar jungles. Flower smallish, greenish-white, March and April; fruit July and August. The *Rohuna Bark* is a useful tonic in intermittent fevers, where quinine connot be had.

লঙ্কা সিজ *Lunka-sij.* A shrub. Coromandel, Guzerat, Deccan, Concan, Bengal, (Serampore,) Assam, Moluccas. Flower small, yellowish, rainy season. The fresh, acrid juice of this plant employed as a blister.

লটকন *Lutkun.* Flower white; immature fruit, green. Cultivated in India.

লতা মহুড়ি *Luta-muhoori.* An annual. Both Peninsulas of India, Bengal, (Serampore.) Flower small, red, rainy season; fruit cold season. *Leaves* and tender tops used in curries.

লবঙ্গ *Luvunga. Clove tree.* Moluccas. Cultivated in Ceylon, the Southern parts of India, the Malayan Peninsula, Mauritius, Bourbon, Cayenne, &c. It has not only not flowered in lower Bengal, but can scarcely be kept alive throughout the year.

লবঙ্গ লতা *Luvunga-luta.* Shrub and climber. Sylhet. Chittagong. Flower middle-sized, white, fragrant, hot season; fruit August and September.

লবান *Luban.* শালাই *Salai.* A tree. Mountains of Coromandel, S. Concan, Jungles above Rajoor, Hill of Shendoor in the Chichooree Talook, of the Belgaum Collectorate, Bundlekhund. Flower smallish, greenish-white, March and April; fruit cold season. This tree produces the gum-resin, *Olibanum,* (কুঁদুরু *Koonduroo,*) a substance chiefly used as a grateful incense, but which also possesses stimulant, astringent, and diaphoretic properties.

লাউ *Laoo. Bottle-Gourd. White Pumpkin.* Annual and climber. Cultivated. Flower large, white, rainy and cold season; fruit cold season. The hard rind of the fruit used as a bottle for containing honey, &c. (*Fukeer's bottles*); a variety of it for making the stringed instrument, called *sitar*; another variety as a *buoy* for swimming across rivers, transporting baggage, &c. (*Royle, J. Grah.*) The fruit of a wild variety তিত লাউ *Tita-laoo*, considered poisonous.

লাঙ্গলি লতা *Languli-luta.* An annual. Manilla, Java, Ceylon. Both Peninsulas of India, Bengal, (Serampore,) &c. Flower smallish, white, rainy and cold season; fruit cold season.

লাল কামলতা *Lal-kamaluta.* Annual and twining plant. North and South America, Mauritius, E. Indies, northwards as far as Deyra-Dhoon. Flower largish, scarlet, rainy season; fruit cold season.

লাল কেশুরিয়া *Lal-keshooreeya.* An annual. Banks of rivers and rice-fields all over India, (Serampore,) Egypt. Flower very small, white, rainy season; fruit cold season.

লাল গুল মকমল *Lal-gool-mukmul.* Flower crimson.

লাল চাঁপানটি *Lal-champa-nutee.* A reddish variety. Fruit rainy season.

লাল ঝাউ *Lal-jhaoo.* A small tree. Soonderbuns. Beds of the Concan and Deccan rivers. Upper India. Flower very small, rose-coloured, nearly the whole year; fruit cold season.

লাল নটি *Lal-nutee.* See কঙ্কানটি *Kunka-nutee.*

লাল পদ্ম করবী *Lal-pudmo-kurubee.* A small tree. Flower double, beautiful rose-coloured.

লাল পেয়ারা *Lal-peyara.* .A small tree. W. Indies, Mexico, Tropical S. America. Domesticated in India. Flower largish, white, sweetish scented, hot season; fruit rainy season.

লাল বাড়্যালা *Lal-baryala.* A shrub. Bengal. Flower smallish, yellow, rainy and cold season; fruit cold season.

লাল বিছুটী *Lal-bichhutee.* An annual. Bombay, Bengal, (Serampore.) Flower small, pale greenish-yellowish, rainy season; fruit cold season. The hairs of this plant sting like those of the common English nettle.

লাল বেতুশাক *Lal-betoo shak.* An annual. Angles of the stem and branches of a fine purple colour; leaves and the mealy panicles somewhat reddish.

লাল বনলঙ্কা *Lal-bunlunka.* A perennial. Cochin China, both Peninsulas of India, Bengal, (Serampore,) Monghyr. Flower largish, yellow, rainy season; fruit cold season.

লাল মুর্গা *Lal-moorga.* An annual. Cochin China, Ceylon. Both Peninsulas of India, Bengal, (Serampore,) Monghyr, Sylhet, Nepal, Sirmore. Flower red or purple; fruit cold season.

লাল লঙ্কামরিচ *Lal-lunka-murich.* A shrub. Flower small, white, and fruit the whole year. Fruit red.

লাল সকরকন্দ আলু *Lal-Shukarkundo-aloo.* Common all over India. Tubers red.

লাল সর্ব্বজয়া *Lal-surbo-jaya.* A perennial. Common all over India. Flower large, bright scarlet, and fruit nearly throughout the year.

লাল সাবনী *Lal-Sabunee.* Plant reddish.

লাল সূর্য্যমণি *Lal-soorjumunee.* A shrub. Peninsula of India, Bengal, (Serampore.) Flower middle-sized, scarlet, rainy and cold season; fruit cold season.

লাহোরী সবু *Lahoree-suboo.* A biennial. Walls, and stony places in Europe. Flower largish, orange, February and March; fruit April.

লিচি *Lichi.* A tree. China. Cultivated in India, &c. Flower small, greenish-white, February and March; fruit April and May.

লোধ *Lodh.* A tree. Burdwan, Midnapore, Nepal, Kemaon. Flower small, lively yellow, December; fruit May. *Bark* much in request as a mordant in dyeing red with *Rubia cordifolia*, L. The red powder (*Abeer*) used by the Hindus during the *Hoolee* holidays is made of the bark of this tree.

লোয়ারি *Loari.* An annual. Bengal, (Serampore.) Flower cold season; fruit hot season.

শকর আলু *Shukur-aloo.* Perennial and twining plant. S. America. Cultivated in India. Flower largish, blue, rainy and cold season; fruit February and March. *Root* tuberous, like a turnip in consistence and taste, eaten by the Malays. No other part of the plant is used.

শঙ্কর জটা *Sunkur-juta.* A perennial. Coromandel, Common in the districts S. E. of Surat, Bengal, (Serampore,) Morung, Saharunpore, Nepal. Flower small, red, rainy and cold season; fruit cold season.

শজিনা *Sujina.* *Horse-radish-tree.* Both Peninsulas of India. Bengal, (Serampore,) Hindoosthan, &c., up to the Himalayas. Domesticated in equatorial America. Flower middle-sized, smelling of honey, January, February and March; fruit hot season. *Root* a substitute for Horse-radish, used medicinally. *Bark*, wounded, exudes a quantity of gum. *Leaves, flowers* and *immature capsules* eaten in curries, the latter forming, a good substitute for asparagus. *Oil of the seeds* in the W. Indies used as salad oil, and because it does not congeal or turn rancid, employed by watch-makers, and for retaining the aroma of delicate flowers.

শটী *Shutee.* See কাখড়া *Kakhura.*

শতমূলী *Sutmoolee.* Undershrub and climber. Ceylon, Bengal, (Serampore,) &c. Flower small, pure white, delightfully fragrant, cold season; fruit February and March.

শন *Sun.* An annual. Both Peninsulas of India, Bengal, (Serampore.) Flower large, bright yellow, rainy and cold season; fruit cold season. Extensively cultivated about Bombay, Salsette, and some places in Bengal for the sake of its fibres, which make a good, strong hemp for cordage, canvas, and paper.

শদি মদি *Shudi-mudi.* An annual. China, Timor, Mauritius, Moluccas. Both Peninsulas of India, Bengal, (Serampore,) &c. Flower small, bright purple, and fruit cold season.

শমী *Shumee.* A tree. Coromandel, Goozerat, Furukabad, Delhi, Saharunpore. Flower small, yellow, cold season; fruit rainy season. *Pods* containing a large quantity of a brown, mealy, sweetish substance, which is eaten.

শর *Shur.* A perennial. Bengal, (Serampore.) Flower rainy season; fruit cold season.

শাড়াগাছ *Shara-gachh.* শেওড়া *Sheora.* Small tree and shrub. Coromandel, Malabar Hill, Bombay, Throughout the Concans, Cochin China, Ava, Bengal, (Serampore.) Flower minute, greenish-yellow, cold season; fruit hot season. *Leaves* employed to polish ivory. *Wood* used for fuel. *Berries* greedily eaten by birds.

শাদা জবা *Suda-juva.* Flower white.

শাদা জাতি *Sada-jati.* A shrub. Banks of the Irawaddi, Prome, Melloon. Taong-Dong, Penang, Bengal, (Serampore, Patna.) Flower 2 inches, pure white, cold season; fruit February and March.

শাদা ঝাঁঝি *Sada-jhanjee.* Annual and twining plant, Bengal, (Serampore,) Ceylon, &c. Flower very small, white, with a yellowish palate, and fruit rainy and cold season.

শাদা নটি *Sada-nuti.* An annual. Much cultivated in Bengal,

শাদা বুড়ি *Sada-boori.* Shrub and twining plant. Peninsula of India, Bengal. Flower none; fruit none.

শাদা হাজর মনি *Sada-hajur-muni.* Peninsula of India, Bengal, (Serampore.) Flower minute, greenish; and fruit the whole year. *Leaves* deobstruent, diuretic, healing. *Fresh root* a good remedy in jaundice. Half an ounce, rubbed up in a cup of milk, and given every morning and evening, will complete the cure in a few days, without any sensible operation of the medicine.

শাদা হুড়হুড়িয়া *Sada-hoorhooriya.* See কানালা *Kanala.*

শানচি *Shanchi.* An annual. New Holland, Cochin China, Moluccas, Ceylon. Both Peninsulas of India, Arabia, Bengal, (Serampore, Monghyr.) Flower minute, white, rainy and cold season; fruit cold season.

শামা *Shama.* An annual. Bengal, (Serampore,) &c. Flower rainy season; fruit cold season. Cattle are very fond of it.

শালগ্রাম *Shalgram.* A biennial. Europe. Flower small, yellow, February and March; fruit April.

শাঁই কাঁটা *Shain-kanta.* A tree. Bengal. (Serampore, Calcutta.) Flower small, white, rainy season; fruit cold season.

শাল শাঁই বাবলা *Shal-shain-babla.* A small tree. Coromandel, Common in Deccan and Kandesh jungles, also in the Sholapore Districts, Bengal, (Serampore.) Flower small, white, rather offensive, cold and hot season; fruit rainy season.

শালাই *Shalai.* See লবান *Luban.*

শিঙ্গাহার *Singahar.* A small tree. Very common about the houses, all over India. Flower 9-10 lines white, with the tube orange, exquisitely fragrant, opening at sunset, and falling off at sunrise, rainy season; fruit cold season. "The orange tubes of the flowers dye a most beautiful buff or orange colour, with the various shades between them, according to the preparation and mode of conducting the operation, but, unfortunately, no way has yet been discovered of rendering this elegant colour durable." (*Roxb.*)

শিবঝুল *Shibjhool.* See নফটকী *Nuphutkee.*

শিম বাত্রাজি *Shim-batrajee.* Annual and twining plant. Peninsula of India, Bengal, (Serampore.) Flower largish, yellow, and fruit cold season.

শিরিশ *Sireesha.* A tree. Coromandel, Bombay, Paghamew, Chittagong, Bengal, (Serampore,) Soonderbuns, Sylhet, Assam, Monghyr, Deyra-Dhoon. Flower small, white, fragrant, hot and rainy season; fruit cold season. *Timber* large, dark coloured, very hard, close-enough-grained for furniture. Large masses of very pure *gum* are often seen on this tree.

শিশু *Sissoo.* A tree. Coromandel, Kennery jungles, Hills about Nagotnah, Goozerat, Bengal, (Serampore,) Assam, Kheree jungle, Deyra-Dhoon. Flower small, yellowish-white, hot season; fruit cold season. *Wood* very strong, greyish brown, with darker coloured veins, but not very durable. Supplies ship-builders in Bengal with crooked timbers and knees. (*Roxb.*)

শীতল পাটী *Seetul-patee.* Mats made of the split stems of this plant, being smooth and particularly cool and refreshing, are well known every where in India.

শুঠী ঘাস *Shooti-ghas.* An annual. Mountains of India. In Honorable Company's Garden flower rainy season; fruit cold season.

শুঁঠ *Soontha.* See আদা *Ada.*

শুড়িয়া মুক্তি *Shooriya-mookti.* An annual. Peru. Flower very large, yellow, and fruit nearly the whole year.

শূকড় টুঁটী *Sookur-toontee.* A shrub. Chittagong, Sylhet. Flower small, white, fragrant, June and July; fruit October.

শুলফা *Soolpha.* An annual. Peninsula of India, Bengal, (Serampore.) Cultivated. Flower small, yellow, February; fruit March and April. *Seeds* aromatic, used for culinary and medicinal purposes.

শেওড়া *Sheora.* See শাড়া গাছ *Shara-gachh.*

শোনালু *Sonaloo.* See বানর লাঠি গাছ *Banur-lati-gachh.*

শোম লতা *Shom-luta.* Shrub and twining plant. Coromandel, Bombay Presidency, Rocky Hills about Loonee. The barren parts of the plain between Dowlatabad and the Godavery. The Kamatkee and Katruj Ghauts; throughout the Deccan, Isle of Perim, Bengal, (Serampore, but very rarely. The late Dr. Carey had only seen it once more.) Flower small, white, rainy season; fruit none. Dr. Gibson mentions, that it is often brought from a distance by farmers, to extirpate *white ants* from their Sugar-cane fields. A bundle of the twigs is put in the trough of the well from which the field is watered, along with a bag of common salt hard packed, so that it may dissolve gradually. The water so impregnated, destroys the ants without injuring the crop. (*J. Grah.*) This plant yields a larger portion of very pure milky juice, and what is rare, it is of a mild nature, and acid taste. The travellers (*Fakeers*) often suck the tender shoots to allay their thirst.

শ্যাকুল *Shya-kool.* Shrub and climber. Both Peninsulas of India, Ceylon, Bengal, (Serampore,) Rajmahal Hills. Assam, Banks of the Jumna, near Delhi. Kheree Pass. Flower small, greenish-yellow, hot season; fruit rainy season.

শ্যামালতা *Shyama-luta.* Shrub and twining plant. Both Peninsulas of India, Bengal, (Serampore,) Sylhet. Sirmore, Kemaon. Flower 5 lines, greenish white, sweet-scented, rainy season; fruit cold season.

শ্বেত অপরাজিতা *Shwet-uparajita.* Perennial and climber. Cuba, Arabia, Moluccas. Both Peninsulas of India, Bengal, (Serampore,) Assam. Flower white.

শ্বেত আকন্দ *Shwet-akanda.* Flower white, cream-coloured, inodorous, or nearly so.

শ্বেত বচ *Shwet-buch. Sweet flag.* A perennial. Europe, Siberia, N. America, Japan. Common in gardens. Flower rainy season. Schultes l. c. is of opinion, that Rheede's plant is widely different from that of Linneus. The latter remarks, that it is the only native aromatic plant of northern climates. The root powdered might supply the place of foreign spices. It has a strong aromatic smell, and a warm, pungent, bitterish taste. The flavour is greatly improved by drying. The Turks candy the roots, and regard them as a preservative against contagion. In many counties in England in which the plant abounds, it was formerly used to strew the floors of houses instead of rushes; a purpose for which its fragrant leaves made it very suitable. The aromatic principle is an essential oil, which can be obtained by distillation. The root has been employed in medicine since the time of Hippocrates. By the moderns it is successfully used in the intermittent fevers, even after bark has failed and is certainly a very useful addition to Cinchona. It is also a useful adjunct to bitter, and stomachic infusions. Thomson (*Mat. Med.* 134) says, it is too seldom prescribed. (*Lond. enc. p.* 257.)

শ্বেত করবী *Shwet-kurubee.* A small tree. Flower single, white.

শ্বেত কামলতা *Shwet-kamaluta.* Annual and twining plant. North and South America, Mauritius, E. Indies, northwards as far as Deyra-Dhoon. Flower white, tinged at base with green.

শ্বেত কুঁচ *Shwet-koonch.* Seeds white, with a black eye; flower white.

শ্বেত কেরই *Shwet-keruee.* An annual. Bourbon, Mauritius, Ceylon, Peninsula of India, Bengal, (Serampore.) Flower minute. greenish, and fruit the whole year.

শ্বেত গোথুবী *Shwet-gothoobee.* A perennial. Both Peninsulas of India, Bengal, (Serampore,) Nepal, Moluccas, China, New Holland. *Roots* fragrant and aromatic. Flower and fruit rainy season.

শ্বেত পদ্ম *Shwet-pudmo.* A perennial. Flower white.

শ্বেত পদ্ম করবী *Shwet-pudmo-kurubee.* Flower double, white, with a yellow throat.

শ্বেত পানী মরিচ *Shwet-panee-murich.* An annual. New Holland, Nepal, Neelgheries, Bengal, (Serampore.) Flower small, white, rainy season; fruit cold season.

25

শ্বেত পুর্ণা *Shwet-poorna.* Flower white.

শ্বেত বসন্ত *Shwet-busunta.* A perennial. Ceylon, Peninsula of India, Bengal, (Serampore,) Bundlekund, &c. Flower and fruit nearly the whole year.

শ্বেত বাড়ালা *Shwet-baryala.* A shrub. Peninsula of India, Bengal, (Serampore.) Flower smallish, pale-yellow, rainy and cold season; fruit cold season. "The *bark* of this yield an abundance of very delicate, flaxy fibres, and might, I think, be advantageously employed for many purposes. When the seed is sown thick in a good soil, the plants grow tall and slender, without branches, and are in every way fit for such purposes." *(Roxb.)*

শ্বেত মাশ *Shwet-mash.* An annual. Cultivated in Nepal, Flower sulphur. In Honorable Company's Garden flower and fruit cold season.

শ্বেত মুর্গা *Shwet-moorga.* An annual. Cochin China, Ceylon. Both Peninsulas of India, Bengal, (Serampore, Monghyr,) Sylhet, Nepal, Sirmore. Flower small, white, and fruit cold season.

শ্বেত রাই *Shwet-rai.* An annual. Cultivated as a field-crop in all the northern parts of India. Flower smallish, brigh-yellow, January and February. *Seeds* used for many economical purposes, especially on account of the oil.

শ্বেত সর্ব্বজয়া *Shwet-surbo-juya.* A perennial. Flower palet yellow.

শ্বেত শাল *Shwet-sal.* Large tree. Circar Mountains, S. Concan, Banks of the Kalinadi river, South Mahratta Country, Bengal, (Serampore,) Khassya Mountains, Assam. Flower small, white, hot season; fruit September and October. *Wood* of the centre of the trunk and large branches, (*Black Wood*) greenish or greenish-black, with lighter coloured veins running in various directions, heavy, sinking in water, close grained, admitting of the finest polish, and universally employed for making furniture. On the coasts of Coromandel and Malabar, the tree grows to an immense size, the trunk sometimes measuring fifteen feet in circumference, exclusive of the bark. In Bengal the wood is not so heavy as on the coast, though equally beautiful, and very much used for furniture. (*Roxb.*)

শ্বেত শিম *Shwet-shim.* Flower smallish. white. Cultivated in gardens and supported by poles, often forming arbours about the doors of the poor people. The tender pods eaten like French beans the seeds never. The plant has no disagreeable smell.

শ্বেত শিমুল *Shwet-shimool. White Cotton Tree.* Moluccas, both Peninsulas of India, Bengal, (Serampore,) Hindoosthan. Flower largish, whitish, February and March; fruit April and May. The woolly cotton that envelops the seeds of this species, as well of those of the Red Cotton Tree, is much esteemed for stuffing cushions and bedding, being unfit for the loom. The *wood* yields a gum, which is given with spices in certain stages of bowel complaints.

শ্বেত সর্ষা *Shwet-sursha.* An annual. S. Europe, N. Africa, Patna. Flower small, pale yellow, February. Cultivated in India on account of the oil of its seeds.

শ্বেত সাবনী *Shwet-sabunee.* Plant pale-greenish.

শ্বেত সূর্য্য মণি *Shwet-soorjamuni.* A shrub. Peninsula of, India, Bengal. Flower white, middle-sized.

শ্বেত হুলী *Shwet-hoolee.* A perennial. Terrest, Bengal, (Serampore,) &c. Flower small, white, and fruit cold season.

সফরী কুমড়া *Suphuree-koomra. Squash-Gourd. Red-Gourd.* Annual and climber. Cultivated. Flower very large, yellow, rainy and cold season; fruit cold season. Flesh of the *fruit*, when boiled, tasting somewhat like a young carrot.

সফেদ গুল মকমল *Sufed-gool-mukmul.* Flower white.

সফেদ তুত *Suphed-toot.* A tree. Persia. Asia Minor. Found in gardens in several parts of India. Flower small, greenish, end of cold season; fruit March. Much cultivated in S. Europe, for its leaves to feed the silk-worm. "Mr. Mutti, an Italian, commenced a plantation of standard trees at the Heera Baugh, near Poona, about fifty-five years ago, on the principle that as soon as they attained a certain size, their roots would strike beyond the sun's influence, and render little irrigation necessary, at the same time that an equal quantity of leaves would be obtained from an equal space of ground, with the further advantage of growing annual crops between the rows of trees. The experiment has been successful, and small plantations under his direction are now gradually extending over the Deccan. One was made in Bombay, near Parell, of about 2000 trees, by Mr. De Ramos, in 1838. It bids fair to answer expectations. The plants are chiefly of the white St. Helena mulberry, to which Mr. Mutti gives the preference from its rapid growth, the small quantity of water required, and the nourishing qualities of its leaves." (*J. Grah.*) Morus alba contains moroxylic acid in combination with lime. (*Turner.*)

সফেদ পুঁই *Sufed-pooin.* A perennial and twining plant. All over India. Cultivated.

সফেদ শকরকন্দ আলু *Sufed-shukar-kundo-aloo.* The red variety is always preferred, and is in general cultivation all over the warmer parts of Asia. Much eaten by the Indians.

সরস *Surus.* A small tree. S. Europe. Himalayas. Flower hot season; fruit rainy season. Leaves and berries are used in medicine.

সর্ষা *Sursha.* An annual. Bengal, (Serampore.) Cultivated on account of the oil of the seeds. Flower smallish, yellow, cold season; fruit February.

সসা *Susa.* Hind. *Kheera.* Common Cucumber. Annual and creeper. Cultivated. Flower largish, yellow; and fruit nearly throughout the year.

সাদা দেবধান *Sada-debdhan.* An annual. Cultivated in India. Flower cold season; fruit hot season.

সাপসন্দ *Sapusund. Sweet Sultan.* An annual. Levant, Greece. Flower large, lilac purplish, sweet scented, cold season; fruit hot season.

সার কচু *Sar-kuchoo.* A perennial. Both Concans, Bengal, (Serampore,) &c. Flower rainy season.

সামদলন *Samdulun.* A perennial. Timor, Java, Lucon, both Peninsulas of India, Bengal, (Serampore,) Khassya Mountains, Nepal. Flower pale red, cold season; fruit hot season.

সাল পাণ *Salpan.* An undershrub. Both Peninsulas of India, Bengal, (Serampore,) Monghyr, Sylhet, Assam, Kamaon. Flower small, rainy and cold season; fruit cold season.

সাল *Sal.* Large tree. Morung, Nepal. Extends more northerly than any other of the order, being found all along the Himalaya, to the neighbourhood of the Jumna, forming vast forests, frequently unmixed with any other tree, but generally confined in the most northern parts within the first range of the hills. Flower middle-sized, yellowish-white, fragrant, April and May; fruit rainy season. It affords the best and most extensively used timber in India; the goodness of which must depend in a great measure on the resin, (called *ral* in the northern, and *dhoona* in the southern provinces) which it contains.

সোলা কচু *Sola-kuchoo.* A perennial. Bengal, (Serampore,) Chittagong, &c. Flower rainy season.

সিঁউতী *Siootee.* Shrub and climber. Deyra-Dhoon, Sirmore. Flower largish, double, white, fragrant, cold season.

সিঙ্গারা *Singara.* See পানীফল *Panee-phul.*

সিজ *Sij.* A small tree. Coromandel, Rocky parts of the Deccan. The Concans, Bengal, (Serampore,) Scinde. Flower middle-sized, greenish-yellow, March and April. *Juice* of the leaves taken sometimes as a purge and deobstruent, and mixed with *Neem* oil, employed externally in cases of contracted limb brought on by ill-treated rheumatic affections.

সীতাহার *Seetahar.* A perennial. Paras, Bengal, (Serampore,) Soonderbuns,) Penang, Singapore, Khassya Mountains. The Ghauts, S. Concan. Flower rainy season.

সুঁদরী *Soondree.* Large tree. Soonderbuns. Flower small, dull orange, March and April; fruit September and October. Used in Calcutta, &c., for fire-wood.

সুখ দর্শন *Sook-durshun.* A perennial. Coromandel. Both Concans, Bengal, (Serampore,) &c. Flower large, white, during the night fragrant, and fruit rainy season.

সুলতানা চাঁপা *Sultana-champa.* Large tree. Both Peninsulas of India. Flower largish, white, fragrant, June and July; fruit cold season.

সুষনি শাক *Soosnee-shak.* Perennial and Creeper. Europe, N. Africa, Mascarenhas Islands, New Holland, Bengal, (Serampore,) Peninsula of India. Flower cold season. Eaten by the poorer class.

সুষনি আলু *Soosni-aloo.* Perennial and twining plant. Bengal, (Serampore,) Flower rainy season. Cultivated to a considerable extent in the vicinity of Calcutta, not only for food, but to make starch of the roots.

সেগুণ *Segoon.* *Teak-tree.* Banks of the Taptee, the Concans, Malabar, Siam, Java, Bundlekund. Flower smallish, white, rainy season; fruit October and November.

সোন পাট *Sona-pat.* *Tinnevelly Senna.* An undershrub. Tinnevelly, Goozerat, about Dholka. Flower middle-sized, gold-coloured, rainy and cold season; fruit February and March.

Leaves milder in operation than the Alexandrian Senna, and occasioning no gripes. The plant comes near to C. Lanceolata, Fork; but is a distinct species, according to Lindley.

সোনা মুগ *Sona-moog.* An annual. Bengal, in a cultivated state only. Much eaten by Bengalies. To be found in every bazar.

সোমরাজ *Som-raj.* An annual. Mauritius, Ceylon, Peninsula of India, Bengal, (Serampore,) &c. Flower purplish, cold season; fruit March.

সোর আলু *Sora-aloo.* Perennial and twining plant. Bengal, Calcutta, (Serampore.) Flower rainy season. The *root* appears to be unfit for food.

হয়ের *Huyer.* Shrub and twining plant. Both Peninsulas of India, Bengal, (Serampore,) Hurdwar. Flower minute, greenish, rainy season; fruit cold season. The *juice of the ripe berries* makes a good, durable, bluish-purple ink. A decoction of the fresh *roots*, with a few heads of long-pepper, in goat's milk, is administered for rheumatic pains, half a pint every morning. It is considered heating, laxative, and sudorific Curry is made of the leaves for patients who are under a course of the roots. (*Roxb.*)

হর *Hur.* A tree. Banks of the Ganges. In Honorable Company's Garden flower hot season; fruit cold season. *Fruit* used like chebulic myrobalans.

হরি কাঁকড়া *Huri-kankra.* Large tree. Bengal, (Serampore.) Flower very large, scarlet, variagated with orange, sulphur and dark purple, February; fruit April.

হলকসা *Hulkusa.* An annual. Mauritius, Bourbon, Madagascar, Moluccas, Philippines, Peninsula of India, Bengal, (Serampore.) Flower eight lines, white, cold season; fruit hot season. Has a pleasant, faint, aromatic smell.

হলুদ *Hulood. Hind.* হলদি *Huldee. Turmeric.* A perennial. Cultivated all over India, where it is much used for culinary purposes. The Javanese make an ointment with the pounded roots, and rub it all over their bodies, as a preservation against cutaneous diseases. (*Rumph.*) Hindus use it as a favorite application to recent wounds and bruises, leech-bites &c. Flower largish, whitish, with a faint tinge of yellowish, the tuft greenish-whitish, rainy season; fruit none.

হলদি আলগোসা লতা *Huldee-algosa-luta.* An annual. Coromandel. The Concans, Mahableshwar, Guzerat, Bengal, (Serampore, Sylhet.) Parasitic on trees and shrubs. Flower small, white, February and March; fruit April.

হলদি বসন্ত *Huldee-busunto.* An annual. All over India. Flower small, bright yellow, and fruit throughout the year.

হলদি মুর্গা *Huldee-moorga.* An annual. Flower gold-coloured.

হলদি লঙ্কা মরিচ *Huldee lungka-murich.* A shrub. Fruit yellow.

হলসী *Hulse.* A small tree. N. Holland, Moluccas, Java. Coasts of both Peninsulas of India, Soonderbuns. Flower smallish. white, fragrant, hot season. Bees give it the preference to all other shrubs, in attaching their combs to it.

হাঁচুটি *Hachutee.* An annual. Java, Bengal, (Serampore.) Flower February and March; fruit hot season. The minute seeds are used as a sternutatory. Roxb. says he often used them successfully himself.

হাকুই *Hakooi* See দন্তী *Duntee.*

হাকুচ *Hakooch.* Annual and biennial. Arabia. Both Peninsulas of India, Bengal, (Serampore) Deyra-Dhoon, Kheree Jungle. Flower small, pale lilac, with the wings and keel dark purple-tipped, cold season; fruit hot season.

হাকুচ কাঁটা *Hakooch-kanta.* A shrub. Sea-shores of India and New Holland, (Soonderbuns.) Flower large, blue, rainy and cold season; fruit cold season.

হাজর মনি *Hajur-muni.* An annual. Peninsula of India, Bengal, (Serampore,) Moluccas. Flower minute, greenish; and fruit the whole year. *Plant* powerfully diuretic.

হাড় যোড়া *Hurjora.* Perennial and climber. Both Peninsulas of India, Bengal, (Serampore.) Flower small, white, rainy season; fruit cold season. *Tender leaves* and *young shoots* eaten. *Berries* very acrid.

হাতশুঁড়া *Hatsoora.* An annual. Flower small, lilac-bluish, rainy season; fruit cold season.

হাতা যোড়া *Hatajora.* Perennial and Creeper. Bengal, (Serampore.) Flower rainy season.

হাতি কানা *Huti-kana.* A shrub. Sylhet. Flower more than 5 inches long, greenish-white, with the mouth of the throat marked with 5 purple dots, April and May; fruit June and July.

হাপরমালী *Hapurmalee.* Large shrub and twining plant. Taong-Dong Banks of the Irawaddi, Bengal, (Serampore,) Sylhet, Hindoosthan, Nepal. Flower middle sized, white, pleasantly fragrant, cold and hot season; fruit cold season.

হাম কাট ঝুলি *Ham-kata-jhooli.* Large shrub. Coromandel, Concans, Bengal, (Serampore.) Flower small, greenish; and fruit the whole year. Wood white and durable, employed by the Hill people for various economical purposes. Cattle eat the leaves. Frequently employed for ornamental hedges.

হরীতকী *Horeetukee.* Large tree. Both Peninsulas of India, Bengal, Monghyr up to Lower Nepal. Flower small, whitish, offensively smelling, hot season; fruit January and February. Fruit, as well as the galls of this species, very astringent and much used by dyers. With alum they give a durable yellow, used on the Coromandel Coast by Chintz-painters, and with ferruginous mud an excellent black, employed by harness-makers for preparing ink, &c. *(Ainslie. Roxb.)* Unripe fruit, according to age, known under the name of *black, yellow* and *chebulic myrobalans,* and thought to be gently laxative.

হালিম *Halim.* An annual. Persia, Cyprus. Flower small, white; and fruit cold season.

হালি মুগ *Hali-moog. Green gram.* An annual. Native place unknown. Cultivated by the men, to whom the grain is of great importance, especially in times of famine. Flower largish, greenish-yellow, and fruit cold season.

হিঙ্চা *Hingcha.* A perennial. Bengal, (Serampore,) Sylhet, Assam. Flower small, white, hot and rainy season; fruit rainy season. *Leaves* eaten.

হিঙ্গন *Hingon.* Deccan, Goozerat, Circars, &c. Flower small, green, April and May; fruit none.

হিজল *Hijul.* Large tree. Both Peninsulas of India, Bengal, (Serampore,) Morung, Saharanpore. Flower smallish, reddish-white, with scarlet filaments, April and May; fruit cold season.

হিজলি মেন্দি *Hijolce-mendee.* A shrub. Ceylon, Peninsula of India. Flower as large as those of the common myrtle, white; and fruit throughout the year.

হিজলি বাদাম *Hijli-badam.* A tree. W. Indies, Mexico, S. America, Moluccas, Malabar and Parell Hills, Bombay, Salsette, Penang, Tavoy, Chittagong. Flower smallish, greenish-red, February and March; fruit rainy season. The *Cashew-tree* annually exudes from 5-12 pounds weight of a fine semitransparent *gum,* like gum-arabic, and not inferior to it in virtue or quality. From the body of the tree is procured by tapping or incision a *milky juice.* which will stain linen of a deep black that cannot be washed out again. The *receptacle* of the fruit has an agreeable, acidulous, sub-astringent flavour, and is eaten like an apple. The juice expressed from it and fermented, yields a pleasant wine, and distilled, affords a spirit, far exceeding arrack or rum. The *Cashew-nut* springs from one end of the receptacle, and has two shells, between which there is a thick inflammable *oil.* This is very caustic, will raise blisters on the skin, and has often been very troublesome to those who have incautiously put the nuts into their mouths to break the shell. It has been used successfully in eating off ring-worms, cancerous, ulcers and corns, but it ought to be applied with caution. The *kernel,* when fresh, has a most delicious taste, and abounds with a sweet milky-juice. When older, it is usually roasted and then eaten as a moderately good substitute for almonds. (*G. Don.*)

হিম সাগর *Himsagur.* An undershrub. Moluccas, Java, Mauritius, Bourbon Hills about Dharwar, Pandooghur Fort, near Wye, Bengal, (Serampore, Patna.) Flower smallish, bright-yellow, rainy season; fruit cold season.

হিল্লুয়া *Hillooa.* *Common Asparagus.* A perennial. Europe. Cultivated. Flower two lines, yellowish-green, March and April,

হুড়হুড়িয়া *Hoorhooriya.* An annual. Both Peninsulas of India, Bengal, (Serampore,) Saharanpore, Nepal. Flower smallish, yellow, and fruit nearly the whole year. *Leaves,* bruised and applied to the skin, act as a sinapism. *Seeds* pungent, used in curries.

হুড়ুয়া *Hoorooya.* A small tree. Coromandel. South Concan, Soonderbuns, Assam Flower minute, greenish. and fruit nearly the whole year.

হোগলা *Hogla. Elephant Grass.* A perennial. Margins of tanks and beds of rivers throughout India. Flower rainy and cold season. Elephants are fond of this grass. It is of great importance for binding the soil on the banks of the Indus with its long tortuous roots, of which great care is taken, when the culms are cut down to make matting of. They are also tied in bundles, and used as buoys to swim with, like *sedges* (Sparganium ramosum, Swz.) in England. *(J. Grah. l. c.)* The pollen of the flowers is abundant in this as well as in the other species, and if a light is applied to it, a flash of fire is produced.
